P9-AOM-127

THE
WELLNESS
BOOK
OF I.B.S.

THE WELLNESS BOOK OF I.B.S.

How to Achieve Relief from
Irritable Bowel Syndrome and
Live a Symptom-Free Life

DERALEE SCANLON, R. D.

WITH

BARBARA COTTMAN BECNEL

St. Martin's Press
New York

THE WELLNESS BOOK OF I.B.S. Copyright © 1989 by Deralee Scanlon, R.D., and RGA Publishing Group. All rights reserved. Printed in the United States of America. No part of this book may be used or reproduced in any manner whatsoever without written permission except in the case of brief quotations embodied in critical articles or reviews. For information, address St. Martin's Press, 175 Fifth Avenue, New York, N.Y. 10010.

Library of Congress Cataloging-in-Publication Data

Scanlon, Deralee.
    The wellness book of I.B.S. : how to achieve relief from irritable
bowel syndrome and live a symptom-free life / Deralee Scanlon with
Barbara Cottman Becnel.
        p.   cm.
    ISBN 0-312-85226-6 (pbk.)
    1. Irritable colon—Popular works.   I. Becnel, Barbara Cottman.
II. Title.
RC862.I77S28   1991   91-22519
616.3′42—dc20   CIP

First Paperback Edition: December 1991

10 9 8 7 6 5 4 3 2 1

One can never complete a work of this kind without relying on the help of others. I welcome this opportunity to thank: Barbara Cottman Becnel, whose skills in research and clarity of presentation will be appreciated by everyone who benefits from this information; Jack Artenstein, whose original idea for the book started me writing; Lynn Willcuts-Unroe, my dearest friend and fellow-R.D., for refreshing my memory with facts when I was too work-weary to remember my own name; Mona Nichols and so many other men and women who shared with me their personal experiences with I.B.S. so that others might be helped; Dr. Alan Markowitz, for the generous gift of his time in discussing medical questions; Michael Seidman, my editor, whose understanding of this subject made his comments and suggestions uniquely valuable; and Nils A. Shapiro, for being at my side with encouragement and support throughout the process, and who does have a way with words.

Contents

FOREWORD

WHEN PEOPLE INQUIRE WHAT your "gut reaction" is to a controversial situation, in return they usually expect a truthful reply. Unfortunately, for some people the reaction that even the mildest of life stresses creates is a gut reaction that paralyzes them and limits their ability to interact in the world.

These people are prisoners of a hyperirritable gastrointestinal system that is prompted into spasmodic activity, creating symptoms of unpredictable cramping and sudden and often uncontrollable diarrhea. For such people the world is turned inward. Everyday, commonplace life adventures take on the aspect of a potential crisis. Avoidance of all stresses, of even potential stresses, becomes these people's lifestyle. Depression and lack of life's zest ensues as even simple pleasures begin to pose the threat of loss of control.

The very events that should spark inspiration and provide both the challenge and driving force to do better become for these people the barriers that they dread approaching. They become limited by their bowels' irritability. Their self-esteem falters. They lose confidence and their world shrinks to embarrassingly basic considerations: How far is the closest bathroom? Do I have toilet paper in my bag? What if I get trapped in traffic and have to go? What if I can't find a seat near the aisle? What if I get an uncontrollable urge during the job interview and my discomfort is viewed as anxiety about my ability to perform the new job, and results in my being passed over?

Irritable bowel syndrome is both a physical syndrome and a state of mind in which the sufferer is forced to endure the physical pain and discomfort of the disorder when it is active, and the dread of its unpredictable reappearance at any given stress when it is absent. There is little freedom from the concern of this problem.

Whether the sufferer has a mild disorder which affects him or her only when placed under the threat of a clearly identifiable loss or pressure, or instead is unable to leave home because he is having ten or more episodes a day, the problem alters and restricts the sufferers' lifestyle in a way that is difficult for nonsufferers to imagine.

Because irritable bowel syndrome involves sudden cramping and diarrhea, it carries a stigma and shame which, although a person may have matured and developed an understanding of the problem, harken back to an earlier age, to a time when we all soiled ourselves, a time of relative helplessness and childishness. It is no wonder that the problem has not been widely discussed. What television coordinator would program a sufferer as a guest to discuss the ailment? Indeed, what sufferer would want to appear to talk about having uncontrollable diarrhea? It is this embarrassment, spawned from experience in mastering our own bowel control on the one hand and the bathroom and associated finger-pointing of unsympathetic schoolmates on the other, that makes sufferers cringe. They must bear the burden of harboring a poorly understood syndrome, as well as the attendant ostracism, both from other people and of themselves as a result of the self-alienation they feel for not being able to be any better themselves.

The medical profession has been slow to recognize the disorder, and the treatment offered has been largely symptomatic and supportive. Often, professionals treat such people with the very same disdain that has been encountered with the lay public.

Unfortunately, the problem is more common than people realize, and the need for real help is great. This work by a skilled registered dietitian makes several important contributions to relieving this suffering. It describes the entity with candor and compassion. It offers a survey of a wide variety of treatment options, and provides a dietary program that offers real control over the symptoms, giving the sufferer new confidence that in itself is helpful in reducing some of the stress that precipitates the problem. More than that, it takes the problem out of the closet into the light of day and so removes some of the isolation that sufferers feel and lets them know that they are not alone. Perhaps that in itself is the greatest contribution of all.

To all those who suffer, here is a chance for renewed dignity and hope, and for the simple precious calmness that comes with knowing everything can be put under control again.

—Dr. David Viscott, M.D.

INTRODUCTION

IRRITABLE BOWEL SYNDROME IS one of the most common and most difficult of the digestive disorders that face physicians and their patients. The condition varies in severity from minor annoyance to life-incapacitating problem. With no definitive diagnostic test or cure yet available, we are left with a disorder that can be extremely frustrating for both the patient and the physician.

Surveys have noted that between 8 percent and 24 percent of the normal population have irritable bowel syndrome; if other indicators of problem bowel functions are included, the percentage is much higher.

In the office practice of medicine, I.B.S. accounts for 40 percent to 70 percent of the referrals to gastroenterologists. For an ailment that was initially described 160 years ago, our knowledge of its cause and the mechanism of symptom production is surprisingly lacking. We do know that fewer than 50 percent of the individuals who suffer some form of this disorder actually present their complaints to physicians, and that female patients outnumber males. Moreover, we know that a large component of the condition seems to be psychologically mediated, with food playing a role in the presentation of the ailment and its control.

The financial cost, as well as the cost of suffering and loss of quality of life, is staggering. Treatment can involve expensive medical testing to "eliminate real causes," an overwhelming amount of medication to control symptoms, and many visits to physicians with frustrating complaints.

Deralee Scanlon, R.D.

Proper diagnosis requires a good patient history and physical examination. The challenge to the medical profession, then, is a well-informed and caring approach to I.B.S. patients. Eventually, however, the patient must take some control of the management of the condition.

The Wellness Book of I.B.S. takes a major step forward in educating people about this ailment, and assists them in beginning to manage the problem. A large portion of the management calls for the patient to be aware of the important role that food and diet play in both the aggravation of—and control of—the problem.

A helpful volume complete with nutritious and flavorful recipes to provide guidance in treating I.B.S., this book will be of value both to patients who are in the care of physicians and the many who are affected and treating the condition on their own.

—Dr. Phillip Mac
Associate Professor,
Stanford University School of Medicine

ONE

A PROFILE OF MILLIONS

YOU HAVE RECURRING ATTACKS of diarrhea, alternating with constipation, that are always accompanied by abdominal pain. You may sometimes experience nausea, gas, abdominal distension, and on occasion, you might notice mucus expelled with your stool.

You are tension-prone and have lived much of your life through measured movements—almost every outing is determined by the availability of rest rooms and by how long it will take to reach such destinations. You avoid long trips and social engagements for these reasons.

You also limit your scope of employment opportunities, since certain positions require that you not have to rush to the restroom with little warning.

You have been known to shun making new friends because you don't want to have to explain your "condition." Worse yet, you typically have spent years traveling from doctor to doctor, trying to get someone to tell you what is wrong.

If you fit this profile, you could be suffering from a rarely publicized digestive disorder known as irritable bowel syndrome, or I.B.S.

And what you have is quite common.

According to Dr. Thomas Almay, Professor of Medicine and Community and Family Medicine, Emeritus, Dartmouth Medical School, "IBS ranks close to the common cold as a leading cause for absenteeism from work due to illness; it is the most common cause for referral to gastroenterologists."

It's estimated by physicians that 14 to 17 percent of the population, or 35 to 40 million people, are victims of I.B.S.—a tally that represents the greatest number of sufferers of any one ailment in the country, according to a study published in 1986 by the American Digestive Disease Society (ADDS).

Of this group, however, only 14 to 16 million with I.B.S.-like symptoms ever see a doctor. Millions of others, perhaps like yourself, remain silent sufferers . . . often for a lifetime.

Why don't you reach out for help? Perhaps you have never heard of I.B.S. and so have no idea that you have a bona fide digestive dysfunction. Or perhaps you are embarrassed by your symptoms.

Health professionals tell us that some I.B.S. patients are afraid that their bowel problems are really psychological problems—a prospect they are reluctant to admit could be true.

On the other hand, you may be the type of person who tends to downplay your condition, opting to behave as if the diarrhea, the constipation, the pain, and the anxiety are something to be tolerated, to be accepted as a way of life.

"Patients who have had a past history of irritable

bowel syndrome are still having the same problem years later; they are just not complaining about it," reports Dr. Frank Dornfest, who is the medical director of the Family Practice Residency Program at the Community Hospital of Santa Rosa, California.

I.B.S. frequently begins in late adolescence, although it can start in middle age. The average age of I.B.S. patients is thirty-five.

Also, with I.B.S. your gender makes a difference.

Women, it turns out, seem to be predisposed to this digestive dysfunction. The ratio of female to male I.B.S. sufferers is widely reported to be approximately two to one, for example. Indeed, 80 percent of doctor visits for I.B.S. consultation are by women. ADDS research shows that the typical age of these women is from twenty to forty.

Mrs. G.L. is an extreme example of one such female sufferer.

During the spring of 1986, G.L., a thirty-nine-year-old employee of a national health organization, bought a new home, got married for the second time, and was preparing to leave for her honeymoon when she was stricken with round after round of diarrhea.

Repeated trips to the doctor brought no relief and, even worse, no diagnosis as to what was wrong. "I was drinking Pepto Bismol because I didn't know what else to do," she recalled.

For twenty years, it turns out, G.L. has had a history of being hit, when she least expected it, with dreaded bouts of diarrhea, constipation, and painful cramps. What occurred on her honeymoon was simply the worst of all such experiences.

And for twenty years she traveled from doctor to doctor, trying to determine what caused her debilitating and sometimes embarrassing symptoms.

Still, determined to see her wedding plans through,

G.L. decided not to cancel her trip, although she barely survived the cruise.

The more nervous she became about the unexpected onset of her attacks, the more often she was visited by the same. G.L. was afraid to venture but so far from a rest room, so she spent most of her trip confined to her stateroom. She became fearful of eating or drinking, lost a lot of weight, and soon was feverish, dizzy, and nauseated, as well as diarrheic.

Eventually, she returned, from what could have been one of the more romantic times in her life, dehydrated and with a blood-pressure reading that had dropped to 90 over 58. Under a doctor's care and facing the real possibility of being hospitalized, she was finally diagnosed by a gastroenterologist as having I.B.S.

These days, G.L. reports that through diet therapy and stress management she has learned how to control her digestive disorder. In chapter 3, *The Wellness Book of I.B.S.* addresses a critical component of that prescription for good health.

I.B.S. IS NOT I.B.D. (INFLAMMATORY BOWEL DISEASE)

Over the years, I.B.S. has collected many aliases. You may have heard someone say that he or she has mucous colitis, spastic colon, and nervous stomach, among other names. The word *colitis*, however, is a physiologically incorrect depiction. *Itis* suggests an inflammation, indicating that the organ is damaged or diseased in some way.

However, if you are an I.B.S. patient you may be tested over and over again, yet the results will consistently show that there is nothing actually wrong with your intestines or colon. What should eventually be spotted by your doctor, though, is the existence of hyperactivity of the intestines or colon, rather than inflammation. This concept will be explained in greater detail later in this chapter.

But first, it's important to dispel the confusion that is commonly held in understanding the difference between the digestive disorder I.B.S. and the diseases that fall under the category of inflammatory bowel disease, or I.B.D. I.B.D. sufferers include persons with both Crohn's disease, sometimes called ileitis, and ulcerative colitis. But for the reasons just outlined, I.B.S. is not I.B.D.

Crohn's disease and ulcerative colitis are chronic, inflammatory diseases of both the small and large intestines. Crohn's disease can involve the ileum (lower part of the small intestine), the colon (large intestine), and other parts of the body like the rectum, anus, stomach, and duodenum, for example.

Ulcerative colitis causes tears in the inner lining of the rectum and colon. I.B.D. can incite symptoms such as persistent diarrhea, abdominal pain or cramps, rectal bleeding, fever, joint pains, skin or eye irritation, delayed growth in children, and decreased appetite, along with weight loss.

Although some I.B.D. and I.B.S. symptoms are the same, as an I.B.S. sufferer you should take some solace in knowing that your digestive disorder is defined in considerably tamer terms.

I.B.S. is categorized as a functional disorder involving the large intestine or colon, which in turn impacts the entire gastrointestinal tract. A functional disorder means that although there is an abnormality in the behavior or "function" of an organ or body part, there is nothing structurally wrong with that organ or body part. In other words, there is no evidence of damage or disease when testing an I.B.S. sufferer, yet the symptoms of diarrhea, constipation, and pain are chronic and can be debilitating.

As an I.B.S. patient, you have a dysfunction present in your colon—a dysfunction of hyperactivity—which leads to a disruption of the two principal functions of this organ. One function of your colon is to absorb water from the contents of the bowel to recycle back into the body; the other function is to carry what cannot be digested out of your body through the rectum and anus.

The I.B.S. irregularity is found in the erratic behavior of the muscles of the colon. Your muscles do not contract in a coordinated manner. Instead, the muscles of your colon contract in uneven spasms that cause food waste to move through your bowel either too slowly or too quickly.

The result: When waste material passes through the intestine too slowly, too much water is absorbed, which produces constipation or small, dry, and hard stools. When not enough water is absorbed, because the waste material is moving through the intestines too rapidly, a watery stool or diarrhea is a natural consequence.

I.B.S., then, is a chronic digestive disorder that can cause severe discomfort and a diminished lifestyle, but it is not terminal or life threatening.

Again, it's important to remember that I.B.S. is *not* I.B.D. It's also not cancer.

DIAGNOSING I.B.S.

If you are one of the I.B.S. sufferers who has sought help from a medical professional, then it is highly likely that you have an arsenal of stories to tell—probably horror stories—about how long it took to accurately diagnose your digestive disorder and about how many wrong diagnoses were made along the way.

One thirty-three-year-old male who has had I.B.S. symptoms for over three years said that at one point he was told he had a rare type of cancer, which plummeted him into a state of depression. He remembers being called in a month later by his doctor, who said, "Sorry, we made a mistake. It's not cancer, but we still don't know what it is."

Another I.B.S. sufferer reports that many a doctor just "looked at me like I was crazy" when told of this patient's symptoms.

One woman who has had I.B.S. for over thirty years says she was sent home time and time again by her doctor with the advice that nothing was really wrong and with the comment, "Just eat what agrees with you."

And yet another I.B.S. sufferer was put on steroids for several years before it was determined that she had I.B.S.

Traditionally, I.B.S. has been diagnosed through the process of exclusion. Typically, depending upon the judgment of the physician, a number of tests are administered to the potential I.B.S. sufferer in order to rule out other, more serious, conditions. These diagnostic procedures can include, among other things, blood and stool tests, X rays, ultrasounds, CAT scans of the pancreas, and a sigmoidoscopic examination—a test whereby a lighted tube is passed through the rectum into the sigmoid colon. A detailed family history of the patient also plays an important role in identifying I.B.S.

Recently, new arguments have been raised about the value or necessity of excessive testing. In fact, some doctors have taken the position that a diagnosis of I.B.S. by inclusion, rather than exclusion, is now possible, with the addition of minimal, selective testing.

Medical director Frank Dornfest of the Family Practice Residency Program in Santa Rosa supports the new findings: "It has been my experience that the most specific symptom associated with irritable bowel syndrome is abdominal pain relieved by the passage of stool or flatus.

"Usually when patients come to you, they have had this condition for a long time," he adds. "So, if you have a patient who presents to you a story that for fifteen years he has been having these symptoms," to what extent is it necessary to carry out an extensive diagnostic investigation? he asked in the *Journal of Family Practice*, Volume 20, Number 2, 1985.

Another well-known expert in the field agrees. W. Grant Thompson, M.D., a gastroenterologist and professor of medicine at Ottawa Civic Hospital, explains the rationale for the new approach to identifying I.B.S. this way:

"Management of I.B.S. must begin with a positive, secure diagnosis. There is now good evidence that I.B.S. can be positively identified by a careful history and physical examination, and that organic disease can be excluded by the same means.

"The cardinal features of I.B.S. are abdominal pain, altered bowel habit, and gaseousness or a feeling of distension. They may occur individually, but when all three occur together, a diagnosis of I.B.S. is very likely.

"There is also good evidence that once established, there is seldom need to alter the diagnosis over time. This is a chronic disease which affects people for long periods of time. It is important that they be protected from unnecessary investigation and overzealous treatment."

As an example, it has been noted that certain I.B.S. symptoms (i.e. bloating, cramping, diarrhea) can also occur from lactose or wheat intolerance. It is important to determine which of these ailments is actually the problem.

Still, many doctors are reluctant to adopt a policy of taking fewer tests because of their own fears as well as those of their patients. Doctors, according to an ADDS report, tend to practice "defensive" medicine due to the number of malpractice lawsuits that exist today. You, as a patient, on the other hand, want reassurance that you don't have cancer or some other serious illness, especially since you have gone so long not knowing what you have, as well as having been misdiagnosed so often.

Also, the notion of relying on fewer tests by definition means relying more heavily on the family history and on simply listening to what the patient has to say—a method that can prove infinitely more complex than just taking a test.

And Professor Elois Ann Berlin, of Stanford University's Family Medicine Division, admits in a paper entitled "Functional Bowel Syndrome, Pheochromocytoma, or Demonio?" that such an approach is not a typical part of the standard clinical interview. Nevertheless, this professor has developed the LEARN model to help doctors and others improve their interviewing skills. And it's a model she employed to make a breakthrough in an interesting case study that involved a young Puerto Rican woman.

Berlin describes her model in this way:

"LEARN: the L for *listen* with sympathy and understanding to the patient's perception of the problem; E for *explain* your perception of the problem, which is normally the biomedical or psychosocial model; A for *acknowledge* and discuss the differences and similarities; R for *recommend* treatment; and N for *negotiate* agreement."

The twenty-one-year-old woman of Puerto Rican ancestry was a dental assistant who complained of a history of abdominal pain and nervousness that went back several years. What brought her to see a doctor was a two-month history of periodic attacks of gastric pain that surfaced as often as two or three times each day.

The patient had started eating less because she believed the pain was made worse by the consumption of food. She also reported alternating episodes of diarrhea and constipation.

For about four months, the young woman saw her doctor on a weekly basis. The pain continued throughout this period, but the severity and location of the pain varied from visit to visit.

According to Dr. Phillip Mac, chairman of the Department of Family Practice at the San Jose Hospital, "She [the patient] was treated with a variety of medications, including intensive antacids for possible peptic problems, but . . . during this time the results of a gastrointestinal series [of tests] were negative, as were the results of a gall bladder series."

A number of other medications were recommended, but they, too, provided no relief of her symptoms. Her pulse rate consistently ranged from 100 to 136 beats per minute during her term of treatment.

Upon a close examination of the patient's personal history, the following was uncovered.

The patient had lived with her parents, as did her two older sisters, aged twenty-six and twenty-four years old, all of her life. She had been raised in a very rigid and religious household. Her mother and father were quite strict. The daughters, for example, including the twenty-six-year-old, had to adhere to a curfew as well as an 11:00 P.M. forced-bedtime requirement. Meals in that household were eaten separately: the parents ate first and the children followed.

The parents did not allow the children to have much contact with the surrounding community. Physical discipline, such as beatings for seemingly insignificant transgressions, was the norm. The patient, it turns out, had been trying over the past few months to break out of her mode of compliance.

Yet the doctor in this case did not jump to make a psychosocial diagnosis of this young woman's physiological problems.

Six to eight months into working with this patient, the attending physicians decided to take a different tack, and made an effort to solicit even more information from this youthful sufferer—information that eventually provided a significant link to establishing an appropriate diagnosis and method of treatment.

The patient's mother had a history of chronic nervousness and irritability. Very often her temper was short—a state of ill health that this matriarch called *nervios*. This condition, *nervios*, was used by the mother to make the children obey. "If you don't behave," she was known to say, "you may cause my death."

As described by the mother, the patient's problem was just another example of *nervios*. And given that interpretation of the illness, the mother insisted that medical expenses and medications were to no avail. With *nervios*, her cultural tradition dictated, there was no cure.

The mother also blamed her youngest daughter's state of digestive disorder and rebellion on demons. According to the mother, both the house the family lived in and her daughter were possessed by the *demonio*. The young woman believed her mother's tale. And though Dr. Berlin did not share the same belief system, she did employ her LEARN model to listen, evaluate, and, of course, learn.

Armed with what she found out, added to what was gleaned from the biomedical methods of testing, the physicians were able to diagnose the patient and help her gain control over her symptoms of I.B.S.

Dr. Berlin explains: "This case presentation provides

a good example of using the LEARN model to comple-
ment the . . . biomedical model. The patient was allowed
to discuss openly the explanation for the cause of the
symptoms the family had used; the *L* in LEARN. The
physician then discussed issues of stress in family relations and her [the young woman's] need for indepen-
dence, the explain part of LEARN; [the doctor] related
this to the cultural context of the family belief system,
which acknowledged the similarity and difference in explanation and why they occur; and recommended relaxation techniques and sympathetic nervous system control,
plus working through the family relations," a form of ne-
gotiation.

What happened in this case study provides important clues as to the skill, patience, and openness required
of the medical profession in adopting the new diagnostic
approach to I.B.S., where an emphasis on really getting
to know the patient, on obtaining an extensive family history, is of critical importance.

As described by San Jose Hospital's Dr. Phillip Mac,
"Treating a physical illness without considering the patient's culture may have significant limitations . . . the
more the physician can derive from the patient, the more
he or she becomes capable of dealing with the patient as
a whole person. Even small amounts of time spent on the
patient's cultural background and psychological makeup
are well worth the effort."

Stanford University's Dr. William C. Fowkes offered
some final and definitive words on the value of obtaining
an extensive patient history when diagnosing for I.B.S. as
well as other disorders when he said:

"Many people we [physicians] see in the ambulatory
setting are not infected or suffering from problems de-
finable in generic or molecular terms. They have problems of living. We are trying, however, to be more adept
at being healers, and much has been written about a

more inclusive model—the biopsychosocial model—as a more useful framework from which to approach the world of healing."

THEORIES ON THE PSYCHOLOGY AND PHYSIOLOGY OF I.B.S.

"My whole life has been stressful," declares P.A., a thirty-three-year-old attorney at a major East Coast law firm, who recently discovered she has I.B.S. "I internalize absolutely everything. I seethe, I stew," she added.

Mona Nichols, who recently moved from southern California back to Canada and was the only I.B.S. patient interviewed for this book who did not mind going public with her story, reports that she was a victim of the "what if" syndrome. "I was full of tension all of the time, worrying about what if I didn't get this finished. Or what if something happened. Or what if something didn't happen," she recalls.

Nichols walked around as if on an emotional tightrope, as if influenced by what she called an "endless adrenaline jolt." She adds, "Tension was a chronic state for me."

G.L., the I.B.S. patient stricken with the dysfunction during her honeymoon, says she has always lived with a lot of fear. "I had medical problems when I was young. I had my appendix and a left ovary removed when I was six," she remembers. G.L. says she recalls vividly how she was afraid she was going to die. That fear of death, she states, has never really left her.

Another I.B.S. sufferer traces her chronic anxiety to her upbringing and the personalities of her North Carolina clan. "Nobody ever tells you what they're thinking in my family. You have to read behind the lines with everything they say," she reports.

In fact, "I get immediate diarrhea anytime I talk to a member of my family," states this thirty-three-year-old professional woman. Yet she admits that she has adopted some of the same familial traits—traits that she also admits contribute to her stress levels.

"I, too, rarely show what I'm feeling. If I were to have a nervous breakdown, I probably would have the calmest nervous breakdown in history," she said.

As an I.B.S. sufferer, your own experience may be similar to the testimonials you have just read of what it's like to live with chronic stress and anxiety. Moreover, psychological histories such as yours and the people who consented to talk for this book have come to be viewed by experts as examples of the typical tension-ridden profile of an I.B.S. patient. One consequence of such perceptions is that questions have been raised by scientists as to whether I.B.S. is, in fact, caused by a dysfunctioning colon, or by a colon that is simply reacting to emotional agitation.

Studies have found that the colons of people who do not suffer from I.B.S. respond in much the same fashion as those of I.B.S. patients. Apparently, the gut reacts to stress in all persons. Hostility causes heightened colon activity; depression decreases colon activity.

But the critical question is, why?

So far, the theories have yet to pinpoint an answer to that query, but scientists have learned much about how the digestive system works.

Your digestive tract, which is in constant motion, is kept on the go by the activity associated with a network of nerves and electrical charges between cells. The resulting contractions and relaxations are what stimulate your bowel to move.

About six years ago, doctors and researchers felt that the "why" of I.B.S. might be tied to the abnormality of intestinal motility, or movement, of the classic I.B.S. sufferer—the erratic contractions of the colon referred to earlier in this chapter. Studies undertaken at that time appeared to show that the colons of I.B.S. patients literally contracted to a different beat than that of their normal counterpart. It was also determined that this difference in rate between contractions was controlled in some way by electrical impulses.

According to Dr. Marvin M. Schuster, Professor at Johns Hopkins University School of Medicine and Director of the Division of Digestive Diseases at Francis Scott Key Medical Center in Baltimore, "I.B.S. patients had been thought to be extremely sensitive to pain in general. However, tests have shown that this is not so. In certain pain tests, I.B.S. patients demonstrated a higher tolerance for pain than did 'normals.' But I.B.S. patients were shown to have hypersensitivity to a particular organ: their colons will spasm at a lower pain threshold."

According to Dr. James Wasco, "I.B.S. is a thoroughly modern problem." This specialist in emergency medicine with the University of Massachusetts Medical School puts the blame on stressful lifestyles which leave people with too little sleep and too little time to relax or eat. There is unanimous agreement among the experts that stress plays an inordinate role in provoking attacks of diarrhea, constipation, and pain.

"The result," he states, "[is] an out-of-kilter intestinal system that produces such symptoms as lower abdominal cramps and spasms, loss of appetite, bloating, and bowel irregularities ranging from constipation to diarrhea."

However, since this digestive disorder has been around for many years, even before what could be termed today's fast-paced environment, the existence of

I.B.S. cannot be laid entirely at the feet of our present-day society that is riddled with tension.

Moreover, stress cannot entirely take the weight for the existence of I.B.S., because recent studies have shown that there are other factors, such as one's emotional state, certain medications, at times the very act of eating, and food intolerances, that play an equally critical role in triggering I.B.S. symptoms.

So what can be said about stress and I.B.S.? Clearly, stress is a significant factor in the life of an I.B.S. sufferer and in the life of this digestive disorder itself. In other words, as an I.B.S. sufferer, you typically have a predisposition for chronic tension—a predisposition that is nurtured by the fact that I.B.S. symptoms themselves cause stress.

And, as I am sure you must know from your own experiences, one of the biggest stress-inducing situations an I.B.S. sufferer must face is getting to a toilet in time.

"Sometimes I had minutes and sometimes seconds to get to a bathroom," G.L. stated bluntly. "I gauged everywhere I went based on where the bathrooms were and how quickly I could get to them," she added.

Another I.B.S. patient pointed out that the dysfunction "colors your life in every aspect. It impacts where you go, how you travel, when you take trips, and even the type of work you can handle," she explained with some distress.

An I.B.S. sufferer who had become reclusive said the dysfunction provoked so much tension around socializing that she had, from her point of view, been forced to adopt a sometimes lonely lifestyle. Ironically, her restricted way of living designed to avoid stressful situations often served as yet another source of stress: "When you have to monitor your food and your drinks so as not to have to run to the bathroom every few minutes, it's difficult to go out and party with people."

Driving the freeways can also pose problems if you're stuck in bumper-to-bumper traffic and can't get to a rest room.

Also, you may have experienced the anxiety that surrounds your trying to sit through a long business meeting, or, equally as traumatic, having to leave the meeting a number of times to relieve yourself.

And, of course, one of the worst fears of an I.B.S. sufferer is this scene: you rush into a public setting and are told you can't use the rest room—that it's for employees only.

Hopefully, you have never had to experience the resulting humiliation and embarrassment of an "accident." To deal with this problem, the state of Maryland has passed what it calls a "Bathroom Bill." Signed into law in May 1987 by Governor William Donald Schaefer, the progressive bill requires that retail establishments employing twenty or more persons make their toilet facilities available to any customer with a medical condition requiring immediate access to a bathroom.

Another area of stress for people who have this disorder has to do with simply not knowing what ails them. Because of the traditional methods used to diagnose this dysfunction, as discussed earlier, many people with I.B.S. take months and sometimes years to find out why they feel the way they feel.

Often, I.B.S. patients-in-waiting live with an even heightened level of chronic tension because their symptoms lead them to believe that they have cancer or some other life-threatening disease. In addition, I.B.S. sufferers have been known to experience stress induced by treatments planned for them that either fail to relieve their symptoms or only do so on a temporary basis.

Many patients also are quick to point out that stress has a broader definition for them than for others who don't suffer from this disorder. Excessive emotional stimulation of any type, for example, is likely to aggravate the dysfunction. In the world of an I.B.S. sufferer, even happiness can incite a gastrointestinal attack just as quickly as a state of depression, anxiety, or anger can cause a dash to the bathroom.

"Happiness can be stressful," reports an I.B.S. sufferer. "I have to watch myself to see that I don't get too excited at times and begin to talk too fast," she says. "Overstimulation of any kind can cause problems."

Another patient agrees. "Any overreaction to anything—being too happy or too sad—will trigger it [I.B.S. symptoms]," she said.

FOOD: FRIEND OR FOE?

For many people who have I.B.S., food is the enemy.

Mealtime—a social occasion for some—may not only lead to a painful and uncomfortable aftermath for the person with I.B.S., but to great embarrassment as well. Often, sufferers of this disorder go to extreme lengths to avoid what they believe is the inevitable consequence of a good meal—pain, gas, and perhaps diarrhea, constipation, or nausea. For example, it's not unusual for an I.B.S. patient who must go on a long trip to simply forego eating for many hours at a time so as to minimize the chance of triggering the dreaded symptoms of this dysfunction.

So, as an I.B.S. sufferer, how valid are your fears about what food will do to you? And what is the relationship between what you eat and your digestive disorder?

Obviously, your gastrointestinal tract reacts to food. But does food provoke symptoms in people with I.B.S.? For years there was much debate and skepticism among the medical community as to whether food caused I.B.S. symptoms to flare up. However, when a study was printed November 20, 1982 in the British medical journal *Lancet*, which found that certain foods did indeed cause I.B.S.-type attacks in fourteen of twenty-one patients, the medical profession's attitudes on this issue began to turn around.

Several years later, in January 1985, another article surfaced on the topic. This time, the journal was *Digestive Diseases and Sciences*, and the study centered around the role fat played in stimulating colonic movement, a trigger of I.B.S. symptoms. The finding: there was evidence which clearly showed that fat does, in fact, cause major colonic activity upon touching the gastrointestinal system's mucosal lining.

Further, Dr. Sidney Cohn, Chairman of the Department of Medicine at Temple University, has pointed out that "the strength of colon response is directly related to a number of calories in a meal, and especially the amount of fat in a meal."

Protein, on the other hand, was found to slow down colonic movement once it reached the digestive tract or once it was absorbed into the bloodstream.

With these two studies and others, investigators are beginning to provide a scientific foundation for what many I.B.S. sufferers have figured out long ago—the intake of certain foods can lead to episodic attacks of this digestive dysfunction.

What *The Wellness Book of I.B.S.* provides is a therapeutic dietary strategy that, together with a diligently followed stress management program, will put you in the driver's seat in dealing with this disorder. *The Wellness Book* will demonstrate that I.B.S., a chronic digestive dysfunction, need not routinely cause you pain, discomfort, or fear.

Remember, your diet is under your control. Indeed,

it's the most easily governed factor that impacts your digestive disorder.

Although I.B.S. is chronic, and there is no permanent cure, a carefully managed approach to eating can go a long way toward helping you control this ailment.

MONA NICHOLS: PROFILE OF AN I.B.S. SUCCESS STORY

"I'm not an old crock, I'd rather think of myself as a delicate flower," explains Mona Nichols with a hearty laugh.

According to this longtime sufferer of irritable bowel syndrome (I.B.S.), she could either see herself as worn down by the effort required to monitor and control her digestive condition or she could see herself in a more attractive light.

Nichols characteristically opted for the latter, more positive image.

Born 385 miles north of Toronto, Canada, in a city called Haileybury, Nichols, sixty-four, remembers that when she was about four years old, she used to awaken her mother some nights complaining of stomach cramps. "I had it [I.B.S.] as a little child," she recalls. "Mother would walk the floor while rubbing my back and telling me it was just indigestion or growing pains."

There were intermittent attacks of painful cramps throughout her childhood, but the digestive disorder didn't really take hold until she became twenty-three or twenty-four years old, Nichols says. Yet, at least thirty years passed before she really knew that she had I.B.S. "They called it spastic colon in those days," she reports.

Nichols moved to the United States in 1959 and became a citizen five years later.

For many years she suffered episodes of diarrhea, constipation, and extremely painful cramps. "I was under constant stress trying to keep up my job, family, and social obligations, while feeling so rotten," she said. "I felt very deep fatigue."

During that period when she was still undiagnosed, Nichols was even sent to a cancer clinic for two years, because her blood count was so low it was believed she might be seriously ill. Eventually, she was put on tranquilizers.

But still there was stress, there was pain, there was diarrhea, constipation, and there was no diagnosis as to precisely what ailed her.

She found no solace with the doctors she went to for help. "Often they think you're neurotic," she said. Nichols admits, though, that she lived in a state of chronic anxiety prompted in large part by her ailment, I.B.S. "You can't be more than twenty feet from a rest room," she said. Moreover, Nichols restricted herself to friendships of long standing, since she rarely ventured out socially because of the disorder. "I stayed on the quiet side in my life to survive," she said.

"I.B.S. is insidious. It's there and you don't know it's there, or you don't know that you can do something about it," she said, moving up to the edge of her seat as we spoke.

Eventually, her I.B.S. condition was diagnosed and she was put on supportive medication. But, as she was soon to find out, drugs alone are neither a cure nor a solution to her digestive disorder.

Several years ago, it was determined Nichols had an eye disease that required she be taken off the medication that had helped her with I.B.S. Her symptoms returned and reached a critical stage—fifteen to eighteen times a day she had to rush to the bathroom to be debilitated by round after round of diarrhea, an extreme I.B.S. experience.

At about the same time, her duties as a branch-office representative for a major Southern California utility changed. Now she was required to talk with the public for prolonged periods of time, with no backup personnel to cover for her when she inevitably had to use the bathroom.

"After two weeks," she recalls, "I had to throw in the towel."

Her company doctor put Nichols on disability. As far as can be determined, with that move three and a half years ago, Mona Nichols became the first person in the state of California placed on disability because of I.B.S.

But fate had one more blow to deal. Nichols's husband received a diagnosis of his own: cancer of the colon.

At a time of personal crisis, Nichols rallied and truly got her digestive disorder under control. A resident of Laguna Hills, California, Nichols started a local chapter of the National Foundation for Ileitis and Colitis. Though ileitis and colitis are diseases that fall under the category of inflammatory bowel *disease* (I.B.D.), rather than I.B.S., Nichols felt that through this organization she could at least receive some support for her own disorder, as well as help others.

The first meeting drew only ten people—eight who had I.B.D. and two with I.B.S. Today, as president of the chapter, she has a 400-person mailing list, and has been scheduling speakers for the group's monthly meeting for the past three years. In 1986, her chapter raised approximately $10,000 that went to research projects involving I.B.D.

She also developed for herself a bland, low-fat, low-fiber diet, and experimented with all manners of stress

reduction techniques, including biofeedback, hypnotherapy, and variations on Norman Cousins's laugh therapy.

"Laughter is the best way to break stress," Mona
says.

On June 21, 1987 her husband died, but she reports
that her digestive disorder remained pretty much under
control throughout his and her ordeal.

These days, she reports that "after flailing around for
so many years and being told, 'There's nothing you can
do [about the I.B.S. symptoms],' I'm glad I didn't listen. I
don't ever believe that there's nothing you can do."

TWO

THE I.B.S.
PATIENT:
A MANAGER
OF OPTIONS

THESE DAYS, YOU HAVE many options at your disposal to help control your digestive disorder. Though a Wellness Diet approach to carefully monitored and healthful meals can prove a critical strategy for minimizing I.B.S. symptoms, there are other areas of your life for which it will be equally necessary that you take firm hold of the reins.

Moreover, I.B.S. sufferers who have been the most successful in controlling their dysfunction are typically people who sought out and experimented with a wide range of treatments available for this ailment.

Biofeedback, for example, is becoming an accepted way to help the I.B.S. patient manage stress. In addition, some patients have reported success using more exotic methods of tension control, such as hypnotherapy and laugh therapy. Exercise is also recommended where there are no physical limitations that prevent activity, and certain medications can provide temporary relief of symptoms.

In this chapter I will provide a solid summary of several of the more up-to-date ways to manage I.B.S. symptoms, but the scope of this book won't allow a discussion of every possible option open to you. There may be others, but a useful way to look at your role in dealing with I.B.S. is to consider yourself in charge and fully responsible for finding the right combination of symptom-management techniques that work for you.

The reward for such diligence is great, because if you are willing to create a daily routine that supports in every way possible a health-enhancing lifestyle, it is possible that you can maintain a comfortable existence for many years to come.

SMILE, SLACK, SAG, SMOOTH

In addition to following this book's suggestions on dietary management, you are going to have to learn how to relax. To that end, you will also need to commit to taking advantage of the many techniques available to monitor and control the chronic tension that characterizes the typical I.B.S. patient.

Though, as discussed earlier, research findings have yet to prove that stress *causes* I.B.S., there is no doubt within the medical community, as well as among sufferers of I.B.S., that stress *provokes* the sometimes debilitating symptoms of pain, constipation, and diarrhea associated with this digestive disorder.

One simple way to ease tension in an everyday situation is to practice what the medical profession calls the "4-S." First, when under stress you should smile and "make your eyes sparkle." Then you should take a deep breath and allow your jaw to hang slack, your shoulders to sag, and your forehead to smooth out. This exercise should be repeated more than once, if need be.

Though this prescription for stress management may sound too easy to be of any value, what it does point out is that your muscles respond to relaxation as well as to tension.

Indeed, your muscles have borne the brunt of much of the stress you have internalized over the years. What happens is this: as stressful situations occur that are not externalized or released in some way, muscular tensions begin to accumulate in small increments.

But with each hit from a stressor, the body makes an adjustment and thus adapts itself to the tension. The process is slow but steady and typically unrecognized in any conscious manner for two reasons: the automatic nature of muscular activity, and the fact that muscles represent the greatest mass in the body, which enables them to absorb a great deal of tension before it's noticed.

So, unmonitored, the brain over and over again sends signals to the body suffering from chronic tension that it should brace itself for trouble. This syndrome is often referred to as the caveman's "flight or fight" state of readiness—a mechanism that was needed to combat potentially life-threatening circumstances thousands of years ago.

Nowadays, the problem is that the "flight or fight" syndrome is induced by more trival matters. In fact, rarely is there a life-threatening situation at hand. So the body and its muscles are quite frequently provoked into a heightened state of tension, with no outlet. And since individuals differ in the way they respond to stress, a particular body function—such as bowel motility or blood pressure—can become more active during periods of "flight or fight," while other functions remain normal.

Moreover, many experts believe that these individual physical responses to stress can become habitual. One result is that the favored response to tension in our muscles may become a permanently overactive response, which could eventually make us sick.

Muscles move the body through contractions. These contractions happen as a result of a network of nerves that are stimulated by electrical impulses that interconnect with muscles, as well as with almost every area of the brain and spinal cord.

Although researchers and health professionals have yet to determine all there is to know about muscle tension, there is one point on which they all seem to agree: sufferers of chronic stress would do well to develop the ability to become aware of unfelt muscle tension.

There is little debate over the fact that such a skill is a key to relieving stress.

THE ABC'S OF REDUCING TENSION

There are many techniques you can employ to reduce tension. Some begin with equipment, such as biofeedback methods, while others rely on medication, such as tranquilizers. A number of techniques, though, require no more than your earnest effort. This is where I'll begin.

Progressive relaxation occurs when major muscle groups are deliberately contracted and then released in order to identify where these muscle groups are located. Moreover, tensing your muscles actually helps them to relax, because a muscle will automatically release itself more after it has been deliberately contracted.

Progressive relaxation produces the best results when it's practiced at least twice a day for periods of about thirty minutes in quiet surroundings—at least initially. This technique is simple, but is useful only if taken up and made a routine part of your life.

Also, in the beginning you should learn this method in a reclining position. Try not to fall asleep when performing the technique, since the point is to gain practice in controlling your tense muscles during waking hours. Later, when you are more comfortable with this method, take your show on the road, so to speak, and spot-practice wherever you may happen to be.

One by-product of engaging in this exercise is that you will become more and more aware of how your muscles respond to stress. Basically, the more you understand what it feels like for your muscles to be relaxed, the more you will recognize the existence of muscle tension.

Differential relaxation is a more selective activity that involves relaxing through "willing" the muscle to let go of tension, without the corresponding tensing. Also, this technique typically takes place at random times during the day in a less protected environment than is required for progressive relaxation during the early stages. For example, it's possible to learn how to relax neck and jaw muscles while you drive. With time, you can even learn to relax muscles that are in use, such as your driving leg or the arm you use to shift gears. If you are having problems remembering to relax, write yourself notes and place them on the dashboard of your car, on the refrigerator, on the bathroom mirror—place reminders along paths that you routinely travel.

When you become adept at concentrating on select muscle groups to cause their relaxation, you'll have the skills to learn how to scan your entire body quickly.

Once you really hone the ability to scan, you'll be able to stop the stress spiral at your command. In essence, you will be able to relax at will.

One way to scan is to become aware of, and direct attention to, each muscle group that might be tense. Don't be disappointed if this process takes a long time to run through at first. This exercise, as with most everything else in life, will pay off if you persevere. Soon it will only require a few seconds for you to scan all of your muscles from head to toe, and to relax those muscles in need.

You are physically active (tensing and releasing) when you employ the progressive relaxation method. To scan, you add the power of the mind to quickly locate and test your muscle groups.

Deep muscle relaxation is an advanced form of a combination of the techniques you have learned thus far—you are aware of muscle locations; you can tell how tense you are; you can readily identify the muscles that are in need of your attention, and you can literally direct suggestions of muscle relaxation. The more you practice this method the more your muscles will relax, because the experience will be impressed upon your memory with each attempt. This phenomenon is referred to as re-call relaxation.

A variation on the deepening technique is to count down, so that by the time you count backward from ten to zero you are completely relaxed. Another way to approach this method is to imagine that you are descending an elevator or stairs. Whatever the imagery, conduct your descent slowly and see yourself landing in the most pleasing surroundings.

Receptive attitudes developed by practicing deep muscle relaxation exercises are the building blocks needed to demonstrate mastery of **autogenic** techniques. Autogenic training, or being self-regulated, is another relaxation method that is used when there are no apparent crises. With this technique you are training yourself to work with the autonomic nervous system, instead of with specific muscle groups. Basically, the autonomic nervous system governs the body's involuntary actions.

Imagery becomes a relaxation technique when you learn how to replace distressing ideas with images and thoughts more to your liking. Like daydreaming, you can "replay" favorite musical passages; you can "paint" or "reproduce" mind pictures that incorporate certain pleasant smells, for example.

This technique is an integral part of hypnotherapy methods, to be discussed later in the chapter.

BIOFEEDBACK

"Until you've been led through a biofeedback session, you don't know how it feels to really relax," reports Mona Nichols, a longtime sufferer of I.B.S. whose story was told earlier.

When interviewed, Nichols described her first experience with certified biofeedback therapist Fran Goodman, R.N., as an "ear-opening" experience.

Nichols remembers announcing to the nurse that she felt just fine. Calm, in fact. Yet Nichols recalls, "When she [Goodman] hooked me up to the machine, the equipment issued this real loud screech because I was so full of tension."

Goodman, who works for an organization called the Stress Center in Whittier, California, says that her experience with Nichols is not uncommon.

So what is biofeedback? It's a method of treatment in which people are trained to upgrade their health by using signals from their own bodies. Physical therapists, for instance, use biofeedback to help stroke victims. Health specialists in a number of fields use biofeedback to assist their patients in coping with pain. Psychologists use this technique to help tense and anxious clients learn how to relax.

Chances are you have used biofeedback yourself. You have used it if you have ever taken your temperature or stepped on a scale. The thermometer tells you whether you're running a fever, the scale whether you have gained weight. Both devices "feed back" information about your body's condition. Armed with this information, you can take steps that you have learned to improve your condition.

When you are running a fever, for instance, you go to bed and drink plenty of fluids. When you have gained weight, you resolve to eat less and sometimes you actually achieve the desired weight loss.

Clinicians rely on complicated biofeedback machines in somewhat the same way that you rely on your scale or thermometer. Their machines can detect a person's internal bodily functions with far greater sensitivity and precision than you can on your own. Often, this information may be valuable. Both patients and therapists use it to gauge and direct the progress of treatment.

Certified biofeedback therapist Fran Goodman tests muscle activity through measuring "microvoltage." She also gathers data on the skin's response to stress, which she calls galvanic arousal levels. (This is what is measured by polygraph machines.) And finally, she determines the patient's hand temperature.

For patients, the biofeedback machine acts as a kind of sixth sense which allows them to hear activity inside their bodies. To illustrate this, one commonly used type of machine picks up electrical signals in the muscles (microvoltage). It then translates these signals into a form that patients can detect: a flashing light bulb is triggered, perhaps, or a beeper is activated every time muscles grow more tense. If patients want to relax tense muscles, they try to slow down the flashing or beeping.

Using the game of baseball as an analogy, like a pitcher learning to throw a ball across home plate, the patient, in an attempt to improve a skill, monitors his or her own performance. When a pitch is off the mark, the ballplayer makes adjustments so that he does better the next time he tries. When the light flashes or the beeper beeps too often, the biofeedback trainee makes internal adjustments which can alter the signals.

The biofeedback therapist acts as a coach, standing at the sidelines setting goals and limits on what to expect, and giving hints on how to improve performance.

Biofeedback techniques used to treat patients were developed only recently. The word *biofeedback* was coined in the late 1960s to describe laboratory procedures then being used to train experimental research subjects to alter brain activity, blood pressure, heart rate, and other bodily functions that normally are not controlled voluntarily.

At the time, many scientists expected that biofeedback techniques would ultimately give us a major degree of control over our bodies. They thought, for instance, that we might one day be able to will ourselves to produce more creative achievements by changing the patterns of our brain waves. Some even believed that biofeedback would one day make it possible to do away with drug treatments that can cause uncomfortable side effects.

Today, most scientists have more modest expectations for biofeedback methods, though research has shown that it is possible to attain more control over so-called involuntary bodily functions than had once been believed. Still, scientists have also discovered that nature limits the extent of such control.

These days, biofeedback techniques are increasingly being used to help persons suffering from digestive disorders. In particular, this method has been employed with I.B.S. patients.

In a study reported during the April 12–17, 1985, meeting of the Biofeedback Society of America, two doctors presented results which showed that an I.B.S. treatment plan including biofeedback methods could produce significant reductions of gastrointestinal symptoms.

An excerpt from the annual proceedings published after that affair describes how Debra F. Neff of the Medical University of South Carolina and Edward B. Blanchard of the State University of New York at Albany set up their experiment:

> For the treatment group, twelve sessions were held over eight weeks. Educational information was provided in the first session and discussed throughout treatment. The use of coping strategies to reduce stress was incorporated in each session. Progressive relaxation training . . . comprised five sessions. The goal of relaxation training was to teach participants to effectively lower their overall level of tension, which was proposed to allow the smooth muscles of their gastrointestinal tract to relax.
>
> Following relaxation training, participants were taught a second self-control strategy—raising their hand temperature. Mastering this skill allows the autonomic response of vasodilation of the blood vessels in their hand to occur. This skill [is] aimed at allowing the participants to achieve an even deeper state of relaxation. Following treatment, participants were asked to rate their overall level of improvement. . . .

The result: 60 percent of the treatment group recorded reductions of more than 50 percent on nearly all of their I.B.S. symptoms.

According to Mona Nichols, her biofeedback therapy "kept her on top" during a very stressful period when her husband was dying of cancer.

Still, before you try biofeedback training, you should discuss it with your physician, who may want to conduct tests to make sure that your condition does not require conventional medical treatment first.

Deralee Scanlon, R.D.

HYPNOTHERAPY

To relieve I.B.S. symptoms triggered by chronic stress, some sufferers have turned to a centuries-old practice: hypnotism.

With this technique you can either employ a hypnotherapist or learn how to hypnotize yourself to help control the pain, diarrhea, and constipation associated with your digestive disorder. However, be sure to consult your physician *first*.

Once you are given the go-ahead by a medical professional, here are a few facts you should know about the technique you have decided to try.

First, you should understand what being hypnotized really means, and what hypnotherapy can and cannot accomplish.

One of the more straightforward definitions of hypnotism was written in 1951 by Bernard C. Gindes, M.D., in *New Concepts of Hypnosis*. In the first chapter of that book he says, "Hypnotism . . . is a method of therapy which seeks to dramatize thought into specific action for a definite end."

A more contemporary expert in the field, A.M. Krasner, Ph.D. and director of the American Institute of Hypnotherapy in Santa Ana, California, offers the following explanation:

> Hypnosis is a state of heightened suggestibility which is characterized by increased relaxation and concentration. People are surprised to learn that there really is no feeling to hypnosis. At least not the feeling which movies and television have led them to expect. Hypnosis is not a mind-altering experience. Rather, it is a relaxing experience and, contrary to popular belief, one is not put to sleep. A person is merely fully relaxed and is always aware of what's going on around him.

Since the American Medical Association in 1958 approved hypnosis training, Krasner and others have used the technique to help people seeking relief from smoking, overweight, and chronic stress, among other forms of behavior. Typically, hypnotherapists such as Krasner will assist a troubled person through these problems with a combination of hypnosis and guided mental imagery.

"Hypnosis allows the mind to vividly visualize a situation," explains Krasner. "And what the mind sees, the body tends to achieve."

According to Krasner, at his institute an I.B.S. patient would certainly be asked, "How might your life improve if you could all of a sudden become a stress-free person?"

Visions conjured up by the patient in answering that question are precisely what the hypnotherapist uses to create the imagery that will help I.B.S. patients change the way they deal with themselves and others. Krasner is quick to add, however, that all this is accomplished without applying force or without a patient having to use his or her own willpower.

The following is a transcript of a hypnotic induction tape recorded by the American Institute of Hypnotherapy. Background sounds on the cassette include sea gulls and water splashing against a boat. As you will see, the tape incorporates much of the relaxation methodology discussed earlier in this chapter.

Sit back, relax, and just close your eyes. In a very few moments you're going to be more relaxed than you've ever known yourself to be. I'm going to mention certain parts of your body, and as I do, I want you to just feel that part begin to relax . . . just feel that part begin to relax. In order to help you to relax, I want you to visualize yourself on a very beautiful, little, white sailboat. You feel the sun warming every muscle, nerve, and bone in your body. The sky is the most beautiful blue you have ever seen . . . just a few white, puffy clouds lazing in the sky, and as you hear the sounds of the sea and the sounds of the sailboat, you begin to feel more and more relaxed. As I mention certain parts of your body, you'll feel that portion just begin to relax, so that in a few moments you will be more relaxed than you've ever known.

Starting with the forehead, I want you to feel all the little frown lines, all the little worry lines in the forehead just seem to disappear. The forehead smooths out, feels so relaxed, and you feel this relaxation coming around the eyes. Now the eyelids seem to become very, very heavy; so heavy they don't seem to want to open. They may want to flutter a little bit, but that's okay . . . just feel how heavy they are . . . and as the relaxation comes down around the facial muscles now, all the little muscles in the facial area just begin to relax.

Relaxation comes further down around the mouth now, and all the hundreds of little muscles around the mouth just start to relax . . . so much so that the lower jawbone becomes heavy and the teeth part. The mouth may even open up a little bit with relaxation as you continue deeper and deeper, relaxed. Feel this relaxation now around the lower jawbone and behind the ears so that all the little nerve endings behind the ears just seem to relax as you continue deeper and deeper, and even deeper as the sounds of the sea seem to say, "deeper, deeper, deeper."

The relaxation goes to the back of the neck now, down around the shoulders—so much tension seems to go to our shoulders. By now you feel the shoulders just begin to relax. You can feel them drop a little. The relaxation seems to go to the backbone now, and as it goes down the spinal column, it seems to go out to the sides, so that every muscle, every nerve, and every fiber in your back just seems to relax.

The relaxation seems to come now to the small of the back and around the curve of the back. This warm sense of relaxation comes to the back of the thigh now, and into the hollow of the knee, around the calf of the leg, around the heel, to the bottom of the foot. And each and every toe just relaxes even more and more as you go deeper, deeper, and even deeper, hearing the sounds of the sea as the little boat gently rocks you deeper, deeper, and even deeper. You are calm, very peaceful, very relaxed. The whole head area and back area seem very, very relaxed.

We are going to proceed to relax the rest of you now. Starting with the throat muscles, feel your throat muscles just start to relax. The relaxation comes down the fronts of the shoulders, down the upper arm, over the elbow, down the forearm, to the hand, and each and every finger just relaxes more and more and more as you go deeper, deeper, and deeper, relaxed on this beautiful, white sailboat, without a care or worry in the world. Just relaxing, doing so very, very well now, as you continue to relax. Feel the relaxation now coming back to the throat muscles, down into the chest and all the muscles and organs within the chest area, feel them just begin to relax. This relaxation continues far into the stomach area, and all the muscles and organs within the stomach area seem to relax. This warm sensation of relaxation goes down into the things, over the knees, down the shinbone, across the instep of the foot and into the foot itself, and each and every toe just relaxes more and more as you go deeper and deeper.

I'm going to let you rest for a moment, but when you hear my voice again you will continue to go even deeper and deeper, relaxed, calm and peaceful. Imagine yourself on that little white sailboat gently swaying back and forth, drifting deeper, deeper and even deeper. Now just relax, deep, deep relaxation.

And as you continue now to go deeper and deeper, you are doing so very, very well I want you to leave that little sailboat, and see you and I standing at the head of a very beautiful flight of ten stairs. These stairs are covered in your favorite color of carpet. We are going to go down these stairs now. As I count backward from ten to zero, each number will take you even deeper and deeper and even deeper. Are you ready to go down these stairs with me? Nod your head please. [Pause] Very well.

Ten; take that first step down. Nine; deeper, deeper. Eight; way down. Seven; deeper, deeper. Six; deeper, feeling very relaxed. Five; deeper, deeper. Four; deeper. Three; going deeper. Two; deeper, feeling very calm. One. At the next number you will enter this beautiful place of peace and tranquility called deep, deep hypnosis. More relaxed and peaceful than you've ever known yourself to be. Is that okay with you? Nod your head, please. [Pause] Wonderful. Zero.

Hypnosis has been practiced under numerous labels for hundreds of years.

In the mid-to-late 1800s, Drs. James Braid and James Esdaile brought hypnosis to the reputable medical forefront with their work in hypnoanesthesia. In fact, it was Braid who coined the word *hypnosis* from the Greek *hypnos*, meaning sleep.

For about the next hundred years, the science of hypnosis saw good and bad days until April 23, 1955, when the British Medical Association reported its approval of hypnosis for treatment of psychoneuroses and of hypnoanesthesia for relief of pain in childbirth and surgery. Shortly thereafter, on September 13, 1958, the Council on Mental Health of the American Medical Association recommended that, in view of increasing knowledge, instruction in hypnosis be included in the curricula of medical schools and postgraduate training centers.

Acceptance by the medical community notwithstanding, the I.B.S. patient should not be lulled into believing that hypnosis can produce a magical change in his or her stress-related behavioral patterns. Explains Krasner, "We can't do anything for a person that he is not willing to do for himself. To be effective, you must go into hypnosis with a positive attitude. You must honestly want to change the habit."

LAUGHTER MAY BE GOOD FOR YOUR HEALTH

One I.B.S. sufferer said that during a particularly trying time in her life she read Norman Cousins's book, *Anatomy of an Illness as Perceived by the Patient: Reflections on Healing and Regeneration,* and watched an hour and a half of situation comedies on television every day.

Laughter, she reports, is the best way to break stress.

The Cousins book, published in 1979, described his incredible recovery from a crippling and supposedly irreversible rheumatoid condition. Cousins, it turns out, used massive doses of vitamin C and "Candid Camera" television segments, along with Marx Brothers movies to heal himself. A professor at the University of California at Los Angeles, Cousins is still active and able to tell his story.

The theory underlying laugh therapy involves the body's immune system. The question is posed: Since it's known that negative feelings and tension can cause an immune system to be suppressed, shouldn't laughter and positive emotions cause an immune system to thrive?

"Over the years I have encountered a surprising number of instances in which, to all appearances, patients have laughed themselves back to health, or at least have used their sense of humor as a very positive and adaptive response to their stresses," reports Raymond A. Moody, Jr., M.D., in the book *Laugh After Laugh,* published by Headwaters Press in 1978.

But can his observations be scientifically proved?

Psychoneuroimmunology is the new field that was spawned to deal with the issue of whether the brain can impact the immune system. So far, psychoneuroimmunology research has concentrated on chemicals emitted by the immune system, the brain, and a number of nerve cells. Such chemicals are called neurotransmitters. What the research has tried to prove is, can a hearty laugh enhance the production of beta-endorphins that help the immune system function even more effectively? Or can a great belly laugh cut off the brain's effort to manufacture an immune-system suppressant such as cortisone?

A study undertaken by psychologist David Mc-Clelland of Boston University to prove this connection ran into trouble because of difficulty in measuring fleeting changes in immune cells. What McClelland tried to do was observe how, through an examination of changes in saliva, emotions such as trust, humor, and cynicism impacted the immune system. A substance named secretary immunoglobulin A, or S-IgA, is found in saliva and protects the mouth and nose from "invaders." S-IgA is believed to play some role in lowered rates of certain respiratory illnesses.

McClelland provoked the desired emotions by showing students either *The Bank Dick* starring W.C. Fields, a film about Mother Teresa, or a harsh propaganda film dealing with Nazi Germany. The antics of W.C. Fields and the heartfelt demonstrations of charity by Mother Teresa did, in fact, increase the level of S-IgA in the saliva of McClelland's subjects. However, the impact only lasted an hour before returning to baseline levels.

Despite sketchy research findings, medical professionals and hospitals alike are beginning to find ways to have their patients benefit from the yet-to-be-proven effects of a positive and humorous attitude and environment.

A humor channel on closed-circuit television is provided for patients at Santa Monica's Saint John's Hospital and Health Center.

New York's Babies Hospital hires professional clowns for its Big Apple Circus/Clown Care Unit.

And DeKalb General Hospital in Georgia has what it calls a Lively Room, which sports walls of bright colors and patterned furniture to uplift patients' spirits.

An I.B.S. patient who has managed to escape any serious bouts of pain, constipation, or diarrhea for the past year says that in addition to regularly watching "Too Close for Comfort," "Three's Company," and "MASH" on television, she has eliminated the violence from her life as much as possible. She no longer watches the evening news and only reads the part of her daily newspaper that reports something other than violent activity.

She also suggests that I.B.S. sufferers "brighten their own corner" by creating a space in the house, no matter how small, that is exclusively their retreat when revitalization is needed.

Again, do not embark on a program of laughter therapy or any of these techniques without first consulting with your physician.

LET'S GET PHYSICAL

Developing an exercise program is fundamentally essential to the maintenance of almost anyone's good health; this is especially true of the I.B.S. patient.

Vigorous exercise is a great tension reliever. It's hard to feel grumpy after a good workout because you are dumping glucose—the body's primary fuel—into your bloodstream and you are secreting substances that can give you what has been called a "runner's high."

However, exercise, like the food management program outlined in the next chapter, must be tailored to fit the physiological requirements of the individual.

So before you take your first jog around the block or

Deralee Scanlon, R.D.

sign up to join the local health spa, be sure to see your doctor and secure approval for whatever sweat-producing activity you have in mind.

MEDICATION THERAPY

Although there is general agreement that the problems of I.B.S. can be truly overcome only with changes in lifestyle and eating habits, physicians must for practical purposes also deal with easing the symptoms distress of patients. That responsibility often leads them to prescribe medication as a temporary answer to meeting specific and immediate concerns.

You will want to get off medication as soon as it is practical to do so. Remember, however, that once the medication is removed, you will be vulnerable again to periodic bouts of I.B.S., unless more lasting benefits have been brought about by genuine long-term lifestyle changes.

As with all medications, these must be prescribed only by qualified physicians. The purpose of the following information is merely to acquaint you with some of the more commonly used medications that may be the drugs of choice from your own personal doctor.

There are five general categories of medication. Each serves a particular function. Often, patients will be required to take two or more types in combination, in order to achieve relief from symptoms while at the same time countering any possible side effects from the medicines themselves.

For each of the drugs listed here, I have commented on some of the potential side effects. Keep in mind, of course, that such side effects only apply in certain individual instances, and are by no means universal. Report any such side effects to your doctor at once.

I. TRANQUILIZERS
(anti-anxiety drugs).

The following act to reduce mental tension and anxiety—a particularly vexing problem for I.B.S. sufferers—without affecting normal mental activity. They are used for a very brief time, and only in acute cases. Note: Some tranquilizers can be injurious to developing embryos. Therefore, a condition of pregnancy must be reported immediately to the physician.

Librium. Alcohol consumption must be restricted. Side effects can include dizziness, constipation, diarrhea, nausea, edema (swelling of tissue due to water retention), weight gain, vomiting.

Xanax. Alcohol consumption must be restricted. Can cause dizziness, constipation, vomiting, nausea, drowsiness, and fatigue. It also increases salivation and can lead to weight gain.

Miltown. Alcohol consumption must be restricted. Can cause drowsiness, nausea, vomiting, diarrhea, dizziness, and blurred vision.

Equanil. (Same as *Miltown*.)

II. BULKING AGENTS.

These are food or chemical substances which act to restore the stool's consistency to a more normal condition in order to facilitate natural emptying of the bowel. In the case of constipation, it softens the stool by bulking it up with fiber. With diarrhea, it changes the stool's consistency from liquid to a semi-soft state. (Note: While some people believe that it is necessary to have at least one bowel movement each day, this is not so. Missing a bowel movement is not harmful on a short-term basis. Normal bowel function can range from three stools a day to three a week.)

Learn to listen to your body. Respond to its needs. If, for example, you feel the urge for a bowel movement, do not suppress it or put it off for "a more convenient time." This can lead to constipation, which in turn may create a dependency on laxatives—and a vicious cycle that alters the body's normal bowel functioning. It would then become necessary to retrain the bowel habits.

Konsyl psyllium hydrophilic mucilloid (Metamucil— see also the section in this book on supplements.) Must be taken with a large amount of water, at least one full eight-ounce glass. A mucilage form of fiber, it acts to soften the stools by increasing their size and water content. For some people, it is an appetite suppressant; therefore, you may want to take this *after* meals, unless for some good reason you are trying to control your weight. Metamucil also helps to reduce blood cholesterol. In certain people, it may tend to cause flatulence (gas), especially when taken in excess.

III. ANTICHOLINERGICS
(antispasmodic drugs).

These block the nerve impulses which are responsible for the contraction of the muscle that lines the alimentary canal—the digestive tube which runs from the mouth to the anus. Thus, these drugs serve to ease a diarrhea condition. They can cause "dry mouth" by limiting salivary secretion.

Donnatal. Alcohol consumption must be restricted. Tablets must be swallowed whole. Can cause reduction of taste sensation, as well as blurred vision, nausea, vomiting, constipation, bloating, drowsiness, dizziness.

Bentyl. Alcohol consumption must be restricted. Take with food or water. Can cause "dry mouth," loss of taste, nausea, vomiting, dizziness, bloating, mental confusion (especially in elderly), constipation, drowsiness.

IV. ANTIDIARRHEAL AGENTS
(narcotic).

The following, *in moderate doses,* are used to depress the central nervous system, thus relieving pain and producing sleep. *However, they can be dangerous—and even lethal—when taken in excessive doses.*

Paregoric (Camphorated opium). No alcohol consumption. Possible side effects include nausea, vomiting, dizziness, drowsiness, fluid loss, constipation, anorexia (excessive loss of appetite).

Codeine. To be taken with water or food. Can cause dizziness, nausea, vomiting, constipation, anorexia.

Lomotil. To be taken with food. Alcohol consumption must be restricted. Can cause bloating, constipation, "dry mouth," anorexia, dizziness, drowsiness, vomiting, swollen gums.

V. ANTIDIARRHEAL AGENTS
(nonnarcotic).

To serve the same functions as the narcotic types listed above, but without addictive properties.

Imodium. Similar to Lomotil in action. Possible side effects include abdominal pain, bloating discomfort, nausea, vomiting, constipation, drowsiness, dizziness, "dry mouth."

Remember: Medication must be prescribed only by a qualified physician, and the dosage adhered to strictly. Report any side effects to your doctor immediately.

THREE

MANAGING YOUR EATING LIFESTYLE

IN THE FOLLOWING CHAPTER you will be guided through a process designed to put you in control of an individual diet therapy program to help manage your I.B.S. symptoms.

To begin with, there are some basic points of information that will help you to better understand the overall concept of *why* you will be eating certain specific foods, and what considerations have gone into the recipes and menu plans provided here. The better informed you are about your own condition, and what you are doing to control it, the better you will be able to care for yourself in unexpected situations such as restaurants which offer limited selections.

In order to make these dietary guidelines as easy as possible to follow, I have prepared a list of foods which are to be avoided, especially at times of distress, and in some cases to be done away with entirely. Where appropriate, I have indicated substitutes which can be used:

rice, cornmeal, potato flour, or arrowroot, for example, in place of wheat, rye, oat, or barley flour to eliminate the possibility of a reaction to gluten (wheat protein).

Such guidelines are the basis of the fifty recipes created specially for this book that include soups, entrées, breads, side dishes, and desserts. These recipes have been organized into a Thirty-Day Basic Comfort Meal Plan to take you through a period when you are experiencing I.B.S. symptoms.

Since it is difficult at such times to maintain a properly balanced diet—an intake of all the food groups and the various essential vitamins and minerals—it is advisable to temporarily include dietary supplements. These will help combat a tendency toward malabsorption (due to a weakened digestive tract), and to promote internal healing. An explanation of some of the most important supplements are included here.

Once you have passed the distress period and are free of symptoms, you will want to begin reintroducing some favorite foods which were on the "avoid" list. Since degrees of tolerance vary widely among individuals, and since a carefully organized reintroduction procedure is necessary so that you can isolate your reactions to various foods, I have provided a suggested tolerance testing procedure—a food challenge—which should tell you a great deal about your own dietary limits.

ABOVE ALL, TRY TO RELAX

The food guidelines presented in this chapter—what to avoid, what to eat—are certainly important and can make a big difference in the way you feel. But they cannot do the job alone; they need your help—most particularly in the attitude that you bring to the table, and the eating habits you develop.

We have already seen how stress, tension, anger, and other negative emotions play destructive roles in other aspects of the I.B.S. patient's life. Brought to the table, they can be devastating. As pointed out in the *Journal of Family Practice* (Volume 20, Number 2, 1985), "The emotional state of fear or anxiety will result in hypermotility [increased bowel movement, or diarrhea]. The emotional state of anger will result in hypomotility [reduced movement, or constipation]."

It is clear, then, that mealtimes must be set aside for relaxed, unhurried eating. No gulping down of half-chewed foods. No concentration of thought on the work left behind at the office. Don't forget what was discussed in the previous chapter. Relaxing during meals is a cardinal rule; whether you adhere to it or not will reflect how serious you really are about adjusting to a lifestyle that can bring you greater physical comfort.

As Dr. Jeffrey Bland points out in *Digestive Enzymes* (Keats Publishing Inc.):

> Digestion takes place in three distinct stages, referred to as the *cephalic phase, gastric phase,* and *intestinal phase.* The *cephalic phase* begins as you first think about a meal. If you are relaxed and relish the food before you, the stomach begins secreting digestive enzymes and hydrochloric acid, which will promote digestion once nutrients arrive in the stomach. However, if you are anxious, hurried, or under stress before your meal, acid and enzyme production will be inhibited, which can result in maldigestion.
>
> The *gastric phase* begins when food arrives in the stomach. At this point specific hormones are released which initiate enzyme breakdown of the foods [and] stimulate the cells of the stomach to secrete hydrochloric acid. For efficient gastric digestion to take place there must be

adequate hydrochloric acid secretion and gastric acidity. . . . Inadequate gastric acidity, due to deficient hydrochloric acid, is a common cause of digestive problems, sooner or later leading to an irritable bowel. . . .

After the food has remained in the stomach for a period of time, it is moved by muscle contractions into the small intestine, the first region of which is called the duodenum, [where] the *intestinal phase* of digestion is initiated. . . . But in contrast to gastric digestion, which requires a high degree of acidity, the pancreatic enzymes (in the duodenum) require a neutral pH for optimal action. . . . The release of these hormones is dependent on the acidity of intestinal contents. If there is inadequate acidity (because of an anxiety state while eating) . . . an inadequacy of pancreatic enzymes and bicarbonate may result. Thus, there is the paradoxical situation of an underacid stomach producing an overacid small intestine, resulting in an impairment of the entire digestive economy.

In short, the body is a finely tuned chemical apparatus. It responds to your emotions and can't be fooled.

There are several simple ways to help yourself in this area. Eat slowly and chew thoroughly in order to break down the food into smaller pieces so that the enzymes have a better start. Try to take a brief walk afterward, both to relieve tension and to increase energy expenditure. Perhaps most importantly, take special care not to overburden an already-weakened digestive system by overeating. Your day should consist of six small meals well-spaced throughout the day. While the *total* amount of food consumed during the day is not to be changed, the timing and portion sizes will play a key part in proper digestion. Poor eating habits, overeating, skipping meals, and eating too quickly all contribute to I.B.S.

It may be helpful to keep conveniently at hand already-prepared mini-meals or snacks of the foods specified in this chapter's special recipes and menu plans; these are for periods of distress. I have indicated those recipes which can be frozen and stored for times when a problem hits you and you don't feel well enough to cook.

When planning meals, keep in mind this biological fact: Fat increases the muscular contractions of the colon; protein slows them down. Since these contractions lead to bowel movement, it is clear that, for example, in a diarrhea condition, the last thing you would want to eat would be a high-fat diet, such as fried foods. However, it would be wrong to assume that a condition could be relieved by switching to the opposite diet—that is eating all protein to combat diarrhea. A well-balanced diet will generally help prevent either state.

In the case of diarrhea, it is vital to replace the lost liquids with plenty of water and a temporary avoidance of solid foods. With constipation, water is again important (to lubricate the compacted stool), as is an increase in fiber.

These are among the reasons why all generally accepted I.B.S. diets are low in fat, high in fiber (except in cases where individual tolerance will not permit high-fiber intake), and restricted consumption of foods rich in lactose (milk sugar, found in dairy products and, to a far less extent, in cheese and such fermented products as yogurt). According to Dr. Schuster, the great majority of patients who experience gas problems from eating bran find that the problems disappear in about three weeks. Aged cheeses, cottage cheese, and yogurt can often be tolerated by I.B.S. patients. Lactaid, a private brand, offers a line of dairy products including milk that contains 70 percent less lactose than regular milk, as well as hard cheese and cottage cheese.

Extremes in food temperature also stimulate bowel activity. Soups and other beverages should be served at room temperature.

THE GOOD, THE BAD, AND THE IMPOSSIBLE

Anyone who has experienced the discomfort of I.B.S. needs no convincing about the importance of keeping strict tabs on which foods to guard against and which are acceptable. To complicate matters even further, some foods which are taboo during periods of stress can become perfectly enjoyable at normal times—while other foods are forever forbidden because they are likely to trigger symptoms at any time.

Since it would be difficult, if not impossible, to memorize a list of "good, bad, and impossible" foods, I have provided below a chart of foods to avoid, which should serve you as an ongoing reference. It is applicable to large numbers of I.B.S. patients, but it is wise to remember that reactions to different foods can vary among individuals. Use this chart, therefore, as simply a valuable starting point; it forms the basis for the recipes and menu plans offered later in this chapter.

FOODS TO AVOID	COMMENTS	SUBSTITUTES
Raw vegetables:	Avoid during distress	Raw vegetable juices
celery	Use stalk to flavor	
onion		Garlic/onion powder
garlic	Can be gas forming	
broccoli	Can be gas forming	
brussels sprouts		
corn on the cob		Baby food creamed corn
spinach		Puréed or well cooked
zucchini		Shredded zucchini
green or red bell peppers		

FOODS TO AVOID	COMMENTS	SUBSTITUTES
tomatoes		Cooked tomatoes
carrots		Cooked carrots
artichoke hearts		
olives (black or green)	High in fat	
lettuce		
water chestnuts		
cabbage	Can be gas forming	
dried peas/beans	Can be gas forming	
mushrooms		Cooked mushrooms

Beverages:		
apple juice	Can contribute to diarrhea	
prune juice	Can contribute to diarrhea	
mineral water		Spring water
citrus juice	Unless diluted by half with water	
alcoholic beverages		
coffee		
carbonated beverages		
teas (black)		Decaffeinated teas

Protein:		
tofu	Can be gas forming	Low-fat or nonfat cottage cheese
ham		
red meat	High in saturated fats	Seafood and poultry
smoked or processed fish		
deli meats	High in fat and spices	

53

Deralee Scanlon, R.D.

FOODS TO AVOID	COMMENTS	SUBSTITUTES
Dairy:		
whole-milk dairy products		Nonfat or low-fat Lactaid milk (or Lactaid caplets or liquid)
Fat:	No more than 3 teaspoons per day during distress	Polyunsaturates (i.e., corn oil, safflower oil) or monounsaturates (i.e., olive oil or sesame seed oil)
saturated fat butter*		
coconut oil or any partially hydrogenated oil		Margarine*
fried, creamed, scalloped, or au gratin		Bake, broil, stew, steam
Raw fruit:		Cook or stew
banana		
grapes	Can be gas forming	
apple		Peeled and cooked
raisins	Can be gas forming	
avocado	High in fat	
strawberries	Seeds may cause discomfort	Blueberries
blackberries	Seeds may cause discomfort	

*In this chart, margarine is listed as being preferable to butter, since margarine contains no cholesterol and less *saturated* fat. However, both contain the same number of calories and the same percentage of overall fat. (Margarine's fat is hydrogenated.) In my own personal lifestyle, I prefer the more natural product over margarine, which undergoes a chemical process.

FOODS TO AVOID	COMMENTS	SUBSTITUTES
raspberries	Seeds may cause discomfort	
cantaloupe	Can be gas forming	
Cereals/grains/ starches:		
wheat	If sensitive to gluten	Rice, potato, corn flour, arrowroot, tapioca
barley		Millet
refined flour products (i.e., white bread, pastries)	Can be gas forming	
whole-grain products		Well-cooked brown rice
Spices/condiments:		Cook with sherry or white wine; alcohol will burn off but leave flavor
black or red pepper		
cinnamon		
nutmeg		
chili powder		
parsley (fresh)	Most other dry herbs are all right	
capers		
tabasco		
tamari soy sauce	Can be gas forming	
cloves		
mustard seed		
grated orange rind		
Sugar substitutes:	Can cause gas or diarrhea	Honey or sugar (sugar can be gas forming)
Mannitol		
Sorbitol		
Nuts: all		Wheat germ

55

On the theory, "Better safe than sorry," you will want to stay away from those foods which I recommend you avoid—particularly during periods of distress. If some of your favorite foods are on the chart, you will have an opportunity to test your tolerance for them later. In this chapter, I will explain a useful procedure for determining the food families to which you may be sensitive.

A word or two of further explanation:

■ I have eliminated red meat entirely from the recipes in this book. While it is true that seafood and skinned poultry are fully as much protein as are other meats, the fact is that a diet of the former enables you to cut down sharply on the amount of overall fat and cholesterol. If you wish, you can put back lean meat cuts after your I.B.S. symptoms have disappeared.

■ Do not fry, scallop, or au-gratin anything while you are in an acute phase of symptomatic attack. These cooking methods add either fat or lactose to the diet.

■ If you experience excessive "bloating," lower abdominal cramps, flatulence, or "too much gas," you will want to stay away from the following foods, which are known to be gas-forming in some people: Chinese artichokes, barley, beans, brussels sprouts, cabbage, coconut meat, figs, honey, kohlrabi, molasses, mulberries, nuts, rye seeds, soybeans, wheat, yeast, and two synthetic sugars—Mannitol and Sorbitol.

■ Raw fruits and vegetables have high fiber content, and therefore may be difficult for some to digest. If so, you can purée or juice them. In the case of citrus juices, dilute them with water, half and half.

SENSITIVITY AND INTOLERANCE

Different people react differently to different foods. This simple fact may read like a tongue twister, but the problem it states has great significance about what you can and cannot eat.

Everyone understands what an allergy is: you eat something that doesn't agree with you, and you get a reaction—for example, the hives rash that some people get from eating strawberries or tomatoes. Sensitivities may be caused in varying ways, but one process is suggested in a report published by the Clymer Health Clinic (June 1986). Research indicates that the stomach wall is an imperfect, incomplete barrier to antigenic material (large molecules) which can find their way into the bloodstream before digestion has broken them down completely. In reacting to these "invader" antigens by sending antibodies to do battle, the body sets up a defense system that is retriggered whenever antigens of the same foods are introduced into the stomach, and thus becomes sensitive to those foods.

Foods which are commonly thought to cause sensitivities or allergies (going from the most commonly encountered to the least) are:

milk and dairy products	beef
colas	onions
chocolate	garlic
corn	white potato
eggs	fish
legumes—soybeans and peanuts	coffee
citrus fruit and related fruits	shrimp
tomatoes	bananas
wheat	walnuts
cinnamon	pecans
pork	

57

A *food intolerance* is an entirely different problem. It occurs when the body lacks, or has limited production of, the specific enzyme needed to break down a particular substance in a food. For example, lactase is the enzyme for lactose (the sugar found in milk). Anyone with a deficiency in lactase will get an adverse physical reaction—such as bloating, gas, diarrhea, or nausea—after drinking fluid milk or many dairy products. Since yogurt and hard cheeses contain less lactose, they are more easily tolerated in small portions when eaten with other foods.

Food intolerance is indeed a common problem; it is shared by 3 to 19 percent of adult whites, 70 percent of blacks, and 90 percent of American Indians and Orientals.

A FOOD-MOOD DIARY

The first step in finding out what combination of foods and stress situations are contributing to an I.B.S. condition should be the keeping of a "Food-Mood Diary." Any inconvenience will be more than offset by being able to pinpoint—and head off in the future—these symptom triggers.

I have suggested here a sample diary format, though you can adapt it to suit your own needs. Note that it provides spaces for you to record the details of *every* food eaten and every stressful situation for a single day, together with any physical results.

Since some medications you may be taking can themselves create side effects, thus masking I.B.S. symptoms, you should consult with your physician before starting the diary, seeking permission to temporarily stop the medication.

Day #							
breakfast	lunch	dinner	snack	Foods Eaten	Time of Day	Symptoms (if any)	Cause of Symptoms (Mood, incident, etc.)

NOW THAT YOU KNOW WHAT HURTS YOU...

Once you have determined from your Food-Mood Diary which foods or lifestyle situations have caused symptoms to occur, you will want immediately to include them on your list of things to *avoid*—especially during periods of I.B.S. distress, when they are likely to create even further discomfort.

Later in this chapter, you will find a list of the foods to be avoided; they are the ones which I deliberately omitted from the recipes for my Thirty-Day Basic Comfort Meal Plan, because, while each individual patient may vary, these "avoidance foods" are generally considered to be irritating during episodes of I.B.S. symptoms.

You will want to add to my list those foods which your diary has shown to be troublesome for you.

GETTING BACK TO NORMAL

The Thirty-Day Basic Comfort Meal Plan in this chapter should help you get through an I.B.S. attack by providing interesting and delicious "comfort foods." After the symptoms have passed, however, you will want to get back to your regular eating regimen, including some of your favorite foods which may be on the "avoid" list.

It is true that foods which have caused a reaction on one occasion may not necessarily be a continuing problem. Once the digestive system has become strengthened, it can sometimes—though not always—be able to tolerate a once-sensitive food. This is especially so if that food is eaten only infrequently. Any food eaten as often as *daily* can ultimately present a sensitivity problem.

There is a specific procedure to be followed for reintroducing foods into the diet after an I.B.S. attack and the use of the special Thirty-Day Basic Comfort Meal Plan. When the symptoms are over, continue the meal plan, starting over with day one, but *put one of the "avoid" foods back into your diet.* (One new food only; by adding only this food you will be able to judge your reaction to it. Otherwise, you may be confused about which of several reintroduced foods is causing a problem.) Include this food in your diet once every four days. If there is no adverse reaction, add another of the "avoid" foods. (I call it a "food challenge," because you are challenging each new food to pass your acceptance test.) Follow this pattern, rotating these foods until you have included the favorites you most want to put back into your eating lifestyle.

If you experience any negative symptoms, you should be able to identify the guilty food. Remove it from your diet at once! The cessation of symptoms will confirm the cause, and it may be that you will have to stay away from that food for many months, if not forever. It's a modest price to pay for physical comfort.

During this period of reintroducing "avoid" foods one at a time, it's wise to begin with small portions so as to minimize any potential reaction. When you have satisfied yourself about the safety of a food, you can build gradually to regular-size portions.

PROBLEM FOODS CAN BE TRICKY

Foods come in "families." Citrus family members, for example, include lemon, orange, grapefruit, lime, tangerine, kumquat, and citron. A sensitivity to one member of a food family could very well mean that you have a sensitivity to all the rest.

For that reason, it is important to know all the close relatives of any food so you will be able to avoid them, if necessary. The following chart will be very helpful to you for this purpose.

FOOD FAMILIES

Citrus:	Lemon, orange, grapefruit, lime, tangerine, kumquat, citron
Banana:	Banana, plantain
Palm:	Coconut, date, date sugar
Parsley:	Carrots, parsnips, celery, celery seed, celeriac, anise, dill, fennel, cumin, parsley, coriander, caraway
Beet:	Beets, spinach, swiss chard, lamb's quarters (greens)
Cashew:	Cashew, pistachio, mango
Mutton:	Mutton, lamb
Bird:	All fowl and game birds including chicken, turkey, duck, goose, guinea, pigeon, quail, pheasant, eggs
Grape:	All varieties of grapes, raisins
Pineapple:	Juice pack, water pack, or fresh
Rose:	Strawberry, raspberry, blackberry, dewberry, loganberry, young berry, boysenberry, rose hips
Melon (gourd):	Watermelon, cucumber, cantaloupe, pumpkin, squash, other melons, zucchini, acorn squash, pumpkin seeds
Mallow:	Okra, cottonseed
Pea (legume):	Peas, black-eyed peas, dry beans, green beans, carob, soy beans, lentils, licorice, peanut, alfalfa
Mint:	Mint, peppermint, spearmint, thyme, sage, marjoram, savory
Swine:	All pork products
Mollusks:	Abalone, snail, squid, clam, mussel, oyster, scallop
Crustaceans:	Crab, crayfish, lobster, prawn, shrimp

Oil:	Soybean oil, peanut oil, cottonseed oil, safflower oil, corn oil
Apple:	Apple (cider, vinegar, pectin), pear, quince
Mulberry:	Mulberry, figs, breadfruit
Honeysuckle:	Elderberry
Olive:	Black or green or stuffed with pimento
Gooseberry:	Currant, gooseberry
Buckwheat:	Buckwheat
Aster:	Lettuce, chicory, endive, escarole, artichoke, dandelion, sunflower seeds, tarragon
Ginger:	Ginger, turmeric, cardamom
Potato:	Potato, tomato, eggplant
Peppers:	peppers (red and green), chili, paprika, cayenne, pimento
Lily (onion):	Onion, garlic, asparagus, chives, leeks
Spurge:	Tapioca
Walnut:	English walnut, black walnut, pecan, hickory nut, butternut
Pedalium:	Sesame, tahini
Beech:	Chestnut
Saltwater Fish:	Herring, anchovy, cod, sea bass, mackerel, tuna, swordfish, flounder, sole, halibut, snapper
Fresh-water Fish:	Sturgeon, salmon, whitefish, bass, perch
Plum:	Plum, prune, cherry, peach, apricot, nectarine, almond
Blueberry:	Blueberry, huckleberry, cranberry, wintergreen
Pawpaw:	Pawpaw, papaya, papain (meat tenderizer)
Mustard:	Mustard, turnip, radish, horseradish, watercress, cabbage, kraut, Chinese

	cabbage, broccoli, cauliflower, brussels sprouts, collards, kale, kohlrabi, rutabaga
Laurel:	Avocado, cinnamon, bay leaf, sassafras, cassia buds or bark
Sweet Potato:	Sweet potatoes or yams
Grass:	Wheat, corn, rice, oats, barley, rye, wild rice, cane, millet, sorghum, bamboo sprouts
Orchid:	Vanilla
Birch:	Filberts, hazel nuts
Myrtle:	Allspice, cloves, guava
Conifer:	Pine nut
Fungus:	Mushrooms, yeast (brewer's yeast, etc.)
Bovine:	Milk products—butter, cheese, yogurt; beef

FINDING YOUR TOLERANCE LEVEL

The most common food intolerances are those involving lactose (the sugar in fluid milk and many dairy products) and gluten (the protein in wheat). Unlike the "sensitivity" foods or many of the "avoid" foods, dairy and wheat will only be problems for people who lack the specific enzymes involved.

For this reason, it is generally considered acceptable to begin reintroducing either wheat or dairy foods after removing them from the diet for one to two weeks. This is different from the other "avoid" foods, which must wait a full thirty days before being reintroduced—and even then, only if there is no remaining I.B.S. distress.

You will want to introduce either dairy or wheat—only one of them—for the same reason that you want to be able to judge any reaction without confusion. When you are satisfied with one reintroduction, you can do the same with the other.

In the case of dairy foods, begin with small amounts of yogurt, hard cheese, or cottage cheese. Lastly, fluid milk. (Nonfat or low-fat are preferable to whole milk, because too much fat is particularly undesirable for I.B.S. patients.) Dairy should be taken with other foods, not alone, and in small portions to your personal tolerance level.

In the case of wheat, try adding one slice of whole wheat bread or cereal (oatmeal, puffed wheat, shredded wheat) at breakfast. If there is no adverse reaction, gradually increase the wheat in your diet to be certain that you have no gluten intolerance.

Note: In the case of both sensitivity and intolerance, it is essential that you read the labels of packaged foods before purchasing them. An examination of the ingredients will tell you whether or not one or more of the "avoid" foods is "hidden" in an otherwise acceptable product.

SUPPLEMENTS

The restrictive nature of an I.B.S. diet during periods of distress can result in an inadequate intake of certain essential vitamins and minerals. For example, the deletion over a sustained period of an entire food category such as dairy foods (in the case of lactose intolerance) will generally reduce the amount of calcium available to the body. While calcium is found in other foods, e.g., broccoli and the bones of sardines, the lower levels of calcium in such foods would require you to eat unusually large portions in order to obtain adequate levels.

For this reason, some supplementation may be necessary—at least during bouts of severe symptoms. In addition to increasing supplies of vital nutrients, some supplements also serve to promote healing of irritated areas of the gastrointestinal tract.

According to an article in the February 1988 issue of *Environmental Nutrition* newsletter, "For some people suffering from I.B.S., less than 1/4 teaspoon of peppermint oil a day can lessen the severity of symptoms. Peppermint oil can relax the gastrointestinal muscles, but it may aggravate heartburn."

Consult your physician before beginning any supplementation program. There may be reasons why one or more of these supplements should be avoided in your particular case; perhaps they will conflict with a medication you are already taking. Or your physician may have a record of your adverse reaction to some ingredient in a given supplement.

The following list of some commonly used supplements should provide a sufficient selection from which you will be permitted to choose. I have listed them in general groups according to the functions they will serve for you. Remember: *supplements do not replace food on a long-term basis.* Do not overuse them, and discontinue them as your condition improves and you return to a more balanced diet.

TO AID IN DIGESTION AND ABSORPTION:

The following help to overcome the body's temporary inability to produce in sufficient quantity the enzymes and other digestive agents necessary to break food down into its smallest absorbable particles. RD = recommended dosage, subject to change by physician. (Note: If condition worsens, discontinue the supplement immediately.)

Pantothenic acid: 500 mg per day. This vitamin, one of the B-complex group, restores co-enzyme A in the intestine. It also helps the body to deal with stress by supporting the function of the adrenal gland, which releases a substance called epinephrine in crisis situations.

Lactobacillus acidophilus or lactobacillus bifidus: one gram, four times a day, in water if purchased in powder form. One of the most important measures used in treating I.B.S. because it inhibits the growth of harmful bacteria, it enhances the benefits of B vitamins and improves digestion. The powdered form is preferred.

Metamucil (brand name): one tablespoon, once a day, in eight ounces of water. A mucilage form of fiber that is effective against irregularity. For some people, it is an appetite suppressant. Therefore, some I.B.S. patients will want to take this *after* meals, unless weight control is an issue. Metamucil may also be taken with juice.

Oat bran: two tablespoons, three times a day, in soup, juice, stew, cereal. Counteracts irregularity. May cause flatulence, but the effect should wear off in about three weeks.

Vitamin B-6: One to two tablets of 50 milligrams, once a day. Helps the body to use protein.

TO AID IN HEALING:

Ongoing I.B.S. distress can contribute to irritation of stomach and intestinal linings. The following can help in a healing process. Use what works best for you.

Vitamin A: maximum of 25,000 units per day. Start with 5,000 units per day; increase only with doctor's approval to prevent toxicity.

Hypo-allergenic vitamin B complex: one tablet, once a day. Systemic yeast problems may be troublesome for some I.B.S. patients; selection of a hypo-allergenic brand, which is yeast free, is recommended.

Buffered vitamin C: 500 milligrams, once a day.

Calcium lactate: one or two tablets a day taken between meals.

L-Arginine: two to ten grams daily.

FOUR

A SELECTION OF 50 RECIPES CREATED FOR I.B.S. COMFORT

"A crust eaten in peace is better than a banquet partaken in anxiety."
—Aesop, *"The Town Mouse and the Country Mouse"*

AT THE BEGINNING OF this chapter, I described dietary guidelines generally recommended for I.B.S. comfort— i.e., the avoidance of highly spiced foods, high-fat foods, and raw vegetables. These guidelines form the basis for the following variety of recipes designed to help you enjoy healthful and nutritious dishes that use home economists' "tricks of the trade" to avoid the blandness usually associated with such foods. (Note: while I have been careful to select ingredients acceptable to most I.B.S. patients, omit any to which you are personally sensitive.)

Included are main dishes, side dishes, soups, breads, and desserts. For each, I have included the number of calories per serving, as well as the percentages

69

of protein, carbohydrates, and fat—important considerations in all healthy eating programs.

The recipes are utilized in the *Thirty Day Basic Comfort Menu Plans* that follow. Don't worry about leftovers; they have been worked into your schedule. The symbol [F] has been used to denote dishes which can be frozen, and for which servings can be set aside for later use where indicated.

It is especially important to keep these recipes in mind during holiday times, when the stress of family gatherings and temptation to overeat are commonplace.

MAIN DISH
Chicken Ratatouille[F]

The flavor of this "comfort food" improves when made the day ahead. Dish also freezes well.

2 (2 pounds) whole chicken
   breasts, skin removed
1½ cups water
¼ teaspoon onion powder
1 (1½ pounds) eggplant,
   peeled and cut into chunks
2 (8 ounces) zucchini, coarsely
   chopped

1 can (14½ ounces) whole
   peeled tomatoes, cut up
¼ teaspoon garlic powder
   (optional)
½ teaspoon sweet basil,
   crushed (optional)

In 5-quart Dutch oven, combine chicken breasts, water, and onion; cover and simmer until chicken is tender, about 25 minutes. Remove chicken from broth, reserving broth. Cool chicken and broth. Remove chicken meat from bone and cut into large chunks. Return chicken to pan. Skim fat from chicken broth; add with eggplant, zucchini, tomatoes, and garlic powder to pan. Cover; bring to a boil, reduce heat, and simmer 20 to 30 minutes or until vegetables are tender. Sprinkle with basil during last few minutes of cooking time.

Makes 4 servings

Hints: This can easily be made for 2 or increased to 8 servings. For 2 servings, use the 1-pound can of tomatoes; your stew will be a little "soupier," that's all. Use peeled, fresh tomatoes in place of canned, if desired. You will need about 3 to 3½ cups cubed chicken and 1½ cups broth.

Calories:	*243*
Protein:	*51%*
Carbohydrates:	*30%*
Fat:	*19%*

MAIN DISH
Chicken, Squash, and Rice Soup[F]

This thick, hearty soup makes a meal.

¼ teaspoon onion powder
8 ounces boned and skinned
chicken thighs or breasts,
cut into bite-size pieces
½ teaspoon garlic powder
1 quart water or low-sodium
chicken broth, defatted
1 bay leaf
½ cup brown rice

2 (8 ounces) zucchini, halved
lengthwise and sliced
2 (6 ounces) crookneck
squash, halved lengthwise
and sliced
2 (4 ounces) patty-pan squash,
halved horizontally and cut
into wedges

In 5-quart Dutch oven combine onion, chicken, garlic powder, water, bay leaf, and rice. Bring to a boil, reduce heat, cover, and simmer 30 minutes, stirring occasionally. Add squash; bring to a boil, reduce heat, cover, and simmer 5 minutes longer.

Makes 5 servings

Hints: This soup freezes well; freeze in portion-size bags suitable for the microwave oven. Then just pop one in for a quick meal.

Calories:	*194*
Protein:	*37%*
Carbohydrates:	*49%*
Fat:	*14%*

MAIN DISH
Pilgrim Pasta*

Old-fashioned flavors served in a very *now* way.

2 cups slivered cooked turkey
¼ teaspoon garlic powder
½ teaspoon rosemary,
  crushed
½ teaspoon sweet basil
1 teaspoon olive oil
¼ cup low-sodium chicken
  broth
2 tablespoons dry sherry

4 ounces spaghetti, cooked
  and drained
½ cup crumbled medium tofu
  or ½ cup regular cottage
  cheese
1 (4 ounces) tomato, peeled,
  seeded, and diced
½ cup slivered Romaine
  lettuce (optional)

In large skillet, stir-fry turkey and seasonings in oil 2
minutes. Add broth, sherry, spaghetti, tofu, and tomato
and stir-fry 5 minutes until heated through. Garnish with
lettuce.

Makes 8 servings

Hints: Look for substitute pasta made with American
(Jerusalem) Artichokes

Calories:	253
Protein:	56%
Carbohydrates:	14%
Fat:	30%

*Contains wheat.

MAIN DISH
Turkey/Mushroom Scallopini

An elegant dish for entertaining.

Vegetable cooking spray
1 pound turkey breast slices or
cutlets
Garlic or onion powder
(optional)
1½ teaspoons margarine

½ pound mushrooms, thinly
sliced
¼ cup dry sherry
Feathered green onion tops
for garnish (optional)

Coat skillet lightly with vegetable cooking spray; sprinkle turkey slices with garlic or onion powder to taste, if desired. Brown over low heat, a few slices at a time, adding more cooking spray to skillet if necessary. Remove from skillet and keep warm. Melt margarine; sauté mushrooms until lightly golden. Return turkey to pan; add sherry. Bring to a boil, reduce heat, and simmer gently until liquid is slightly reduced. Arrange on serving platter and garnish with feathered green onion.

Makes 4 servings

Hints: Minced green onion adds good flavor to this dish. Sauté onion and remove before browning turkey; add to skillet along with turkey when adding sherry.

Calories:	*218*
Protein:	*64%*
Carbohydrates:	*6%*
Fat:	*30%*

MAIN DISH
Sonoma Chicken Salad with Ginger Peach Dressing

California healthy and beautiful.

1 (1 pound) whole chicken breast, skinned
3 cups low-sodium chicken broth, defatted
¼ teaspoon onion powder
¼ teaspoon salt
½ cup white rice
1 cup brown rice
1 (8 ounces) cucumber, peeled and diced

5 (1¼ pounds) plums, peeled and sliced
½ teaspoon dry mustard (optional)
¼ teaspoon ground ginger
1½ teaspoon cornstarch
2 tablespoons dry sherry
1 can (12 ounces) peach nectar
Romaine leaves to hold chicken mixture

Trim excess fat from chicken. In large skillet, bring broth, onion powder, and salt to a boil. Add white and brown rice and place chicken on top. Reduce heat, cover, and simmer 30 minutes until rice is tender and chicken is cooked. Add cucumber the last 5 minutes. Cool. Shred chicken. Combine chicken, rice, and cucumber; chill. In small saucepan, combine remaining ingredients except Romaine. Bring to a boil, stirring constantly; chill. Place chicken mixture on bed of Romaine. Spoon dressing over salad.

Makes 6 servings

Hints: To remove fat from canned broth, refrigerate several hours and fat will form an easy-to-remove ball.

Calories: 278
Protein: 19%
Carbohydrates: 69%
Fat: 12%

MAIN DISH
Tuna Soufflé

A soufflé is a little more work to prepare than most casseroles, but the light, tender texture makes it definitely worthwhile.

Vegetable cooking spray
20 small mushrooms
¼ teaspoon onion powder
¼ teaspoon paprika
1 teaspoon dry mustard
   (optional)
½ cup low-fat Lactaid milk
½ cup water

1½ cups fresh rice bread
   crumbs, divided
1 can (7 ounces) water-packed
   tuna, drained and flaked
1 tablespoon margarine,
   melted
3 egg whites

Preheat oven to 350°F. Coat 8″ × 8″ × 2″ baking dish with cooking spray. Coat large saucepan with cooking spray. Over medium-high heat, stir-fry mushrooms for 3 minutes. Add seasonings, milk, water, 1 cup crumbs and tuna and heat through. Lightly combine remaining ½ cup bread crumbs with margarine. In medium glass or metal bowl, beat whites until soft peaks form. Gently fold into tuna mixture so as not to reduce volume. Spoon into baking dish. Sprinkle with buttered crumbs. Bake 50 minutes or until puffy and golden brown. A table knife inserted in center should come out clean.

Makes 4 servings

Calories:	242
Protein:	34%
Carbohydrates:	46%
Fat:	20%

MAIN DISH
Chicken Fajitas

The latest trend in Mexican cuisine, although some say it was a Texas invention.

2 (2 pounds) whole chicken breasts, split
1 teaspoon onion powder
½ teaspoon garlic powder
2 tablespoons lime juice
8 corn tortillas, warmed

¼ cup plain low-fat yogurt
¼ cup mild salsa
½ cup peeled and chopped tomato
Vegetable cooking spray

Bone and skin chicken. Trim excess fat. Slice into ½" strips. In medium bowl, combine onion and garlic powders and juice. Add chicken and toss to season evenly; refrigerate 30 minutes. Prepare remaining ingredients. Coat heavy 10" skillet with cooking spray. Stir-fry chicken, one half at a time, 2 to 3 minutes until browned and cooked through. Place chicken on tortilla, top with remaining ingredients.

Makes 4 servings

Hints: Serve sizzling hot. The skillet may be brought to the table so that each person can assemble their own fajita.

Calories:	304
Protein:	42%
Carbohydrates:	39%
Fat:	19%

MAIN DISH

Tarragon Roasted Chicken in a Bag with Herb Gravy

Casual dining or elegant entertaining, this recipe is always perfect . . . and easy.

Vegetable cooking spray
3 teaspoons tarragon leaves
¼ teaspoon garlic powder
1 (4 pounds) roasting chicken, without skin
1 can (10½ ounces) low-sodium chicken broth, defatted

¼ cup dry white wine
2 tablespoons cornstarch
¼ teaspoon salt

Preheat oven to 400°F. Combine tarragon and garlic powder. Rub meat with half of seasonings. Rub cavity with remaining seasoning. Fold wings under back. Tie legs together. Place breast side up in baking bag, and place in baking dish. Bake 1 hour or until juices run clear when cut between drumstick and body. Remove from bag; keep warm. In small saucepan, combine drippings with remaining ingredients. Bring to a boil, stirring constantly. Slice chicken and place on small, heated platter. Pass herb gravy separately.

Makes 8 servings

Note: This entree is slightly above the recommended 30% level of fat-from-calories. However, this can be balanced by the rest of the day's meals.

Deralee Scanlon, R.D.

Calories:	235
Protein:	60%
Carbohydrates:	6%
Fat:	34%

MAIN DISH
Roasted Game Birds with Mushroom Cream [F]

An elegant, yet simple presentation of any game bird.

2 (2½ pounds) Rock Cornish game hens
Vegetable cooking spray
1 pound small button mushrooms
½ cup red vermouth or low-sodium chicken broth
½ cup water
¼ teaspoon onion powder
¼ teaspoon garlic powder
¼ cup plain low-fat yogurt
Rice or pasta (optional)

With heavy knife or poultry shears, cut birds in half from neck to tail. Discard skin and wings. Trim excess fat. Coat heavy skillet with cooking spray. Over medium-high heat, brown birds on all sides. Add mushrooms, vermouth, water, and seasonings. Cover and simmer 20 to 30 minutes. Remove birds to heated platter and keep warm. Cook sauce over medium-high heat until reduced to ½ cup. Remove sauce from heat and whisk in yogurt. Serve with rice or pasta if desired. Serve mushroom cream on the side.

Makes 4 servings

Calories:	401
Protein:	46%
Carbohydrates:	29%
Fat:	25%

MAIN DISH
Flounder with Rosy Shrimp Sauce[F]

The foundation for an elegant meal.

8 (1¼ pounds) small whole
  flounder fillets
2 tablespoons lemon juice
¼ cup potato starch
2 eggs, well beaten
¼ cup low-fat Lactaid milk, or
  water

¾ cup fresh rice bread crumbs
Vegetable cooking spray
Dill sprigs and lemon wedges
  for garnish (optional)
Rosy shrimp sauce

Sprinkle flounder with juice. In plastic bag, place potato starch and fillets and shake to coat. In flat bowl, combine egg and milk. Dip fish in egg mixture and then in bread crumbs. Coat heavy skillet with cooking spray. Over medium heat cook fish for 3 minutes per side until golden and fish flakes easily with fork. Lightly coat top side of fish with cooking spray before turning. Garnish with dill and lemon wedges if desired. Serve with Rosy Shrimp Sauce.

Makes 4 servings

Hints: When breading fish, be sure to shake off excess flour or egg before going on to next step. When cooking fish, keep the thickest part to the center of the skillet.

Rosy Shrimp Sauce

½ pound tiny shrimp, cooked,
  or 2 cans (4½ ounces each)
  small shrimp, drained
2 tablespoons light
  mayonnaise

¼ cup plain low-fat yogurt
1 tablespoon ketchup
1 tablespoon dry sherry,
  boiled (optional)

Combine all ingredients and refrigerate until serving.

Makes 1 cup

Calories:	*335*
Protein:	*45%*
Carbohydrates:	*39%*
Fat:	*16%*

MAIN DISH
Mediterranean Bouillabaisse[F]

Take a dinner tray out on the patio, close your eyes, and imagine a sea breeze.

1 bottle (8 ounces) clam juice
1 can (10½ ounces) low-sodium chicken broth, defatted
2 (8 ounces) carrots, sliced diagonally
1 teaspoon onion powder
½ teaspoon garlic powder
1 bay leaf
1 can (15 ounces) tomato sauce

2 tablespoons lemon juice
12 ounces white fish (snapper, cod, halibut, or sole), cut into bite-size pieces
8 clams in shell, scrubbed
4 ounces small cooked shrimp
1 can (5½ ounces) shoestring beets, drained

In 5-quart Dutch oven, combine clam juice, broth, carrots, and seasonings. Bring to a boil, reduce heat, cover, and simmer until carrots are tender. Discard bay leaf. Add tomato sauce and juice. Return to a boil. Add white fish and clams; reduce heat and simmer 4 minutes. Add shrimp and beets and continue simmering 3 minutes longer until fish flakes and clam shells open.

Makes 4 servings

Hints: Fresh, live clams should have tightly closed shells; discard any that are open. After cooking, all clam shells should be open; discard any that are still closed.

Calories: 214
Protein: 56%
Carbohydrates: 34%
Fat: 10%

MAIN DISH
Herbed Oven-fried Fish Fillets[F]

Easy, low-cal, and no mess!

Vegetable cooking spray
½ cup cornmeal
½ teaspoon dill weed
½ teaspoon paprika
1 egg, beaten
2 tablespoons low-fat Lactaid milk, or water
4 (1 pound) large white fish fillets (cod, halibut, sole, red snapper)

1 tablespoon margarine, melted
4 lemon wedges dipped in paprika for garnish (optional)

Preheat oven to 350°F. Coat 15″ × 10″ jelly roll pan with cooking spray. In plastic bag, combine cornmeal and seasonings. In shallow bowl, combine egg and milk. Dip fish in egg mixture and then into cornmeal mixture; shake to coat. Place on pan. Drizzle with margarine. Bake 15 to 20 minutes until golden brown and fish flakes easily with fork. Garnish with lemon wedges if desired.

Makes 4 servings

Calories:	*189*
Protein:	*51%*
Carbohydrates:	*25%*
Fat:	*24%*

MAIN DISH
Lemon - Herbed Roast Turkey[F]

A no-mess method to enjoy a delicious roast turkey. You'll enjoy the subtle lemony aroma and flavor.

1 (2 to 3 pound) turkey breast, skinned
1 small lemon
¼ teaspoon sage
¼ teaspoon rosemary, crushed
¼ teaspoon oregano
1 cook-in bag
Rice or whipped potatoes (optional)

Preheat oven to 325°F. Cut pocket horizontally in breast large enough for lemon. With fork, prick surface of lemon several times. Combine seasonings and rub in pocket and over top of breast. Place lemon in pocket; skewer closed. Place turkey in bag; tie bag securely closed. Make six ½-inch slits in top of bag to allow steam to escape. Place in 12″ × 9″ × 2″ baking dish. Bake 1¼ hours or until meat thermometer placed in thickest part, without touching bone, reaches 170°F or until juices run clear. Serve with rice or potatoes if desired.

Makes 8 servings

Hints: Serve with traditional accompaniments or break out and try new and unusual dishes.

Calories:	*275*
Protein:	*48%*
Carbohydrates:	*35%*
Fat:	*17%*

MAIN DISH
Fish Florentine Wrap-ups[F]

Always attractive, this dish works well on a buffet.

Vegetable cooking spray
4 (⅔ pound) thin fillets of
   flounder
1 package (10 ounces) frozen
   chopped spinach, thawed
½ teaspoon onion powder

2 teaspoons sweet basil
¼ cup dry white wine or
   water
1 tablespoon lemon juice
½ teaspoon paprika
1 teaspoon dill weed

Preheat oven to 350°F. Coat 8" × 8" × 2" baking dish with cooking spray. Press thicker portions of flounder to flatten. Press excess moisture from spinach. In medium bowl, combine spinach, onion powder, and basil; spread ⅓ cup on each fillet. Roll up and fasten with toothpicks. Place roll-ups in baking dish. Combine wine and juice and pour over fillets. Sprinkle with paprika and dill. Cover and bake 25 minutes or until fish flakes easily with fork.

Makes 4 servings

Calories:	72
Protein:	78%
Carbohydrates:	14%
Fat:	8%

MAIN DISH
Scallops a la Maison*

As elegant as this sounds, it can be prepared in just 15 minutes.

1 tablespoon margarine
½ cup dry white wine
½ teaspoon onion powder
¼ teaspoon garlic powder
1 pound scallops
1 can (14 ounces) whole peeled tomatoes, drained and cut into pieces
1 teaspoon dried cilantro, crushed

2 teaspoons cornstarch
½ cup low-fat Lactaid milk
2 cups cooked rice or pasta (optional)*
Fresh cilantro sprigs for garnish (optional)

In medium skillet, combine margarine, wine, onion and garlic powders, and scallops. Bring to a boil, reduce heat, cover, and simmer 3 minutes. With slotted spoon remove scallops and keep warm. Boil cooking liquid until reduced to ¼ cup. Add tomatoes and cilantro and simmer 3 minutes longer. Combine cornstarch and milk and whisk into wine mixture. Cook until sauce boils, stirring constantly. Return scallops to pan and heat through; do not boil. Serve over rice and garnish with cilantro sprigs if desired.

*Contains wheat, if pasta is used.

89

Makes 4 servings

Hints: The scallops we eat are actually the muscle that controls the shell. They are very tender, so be careful not to overcook them.

Calories:	*256*
Protein:	*34%*
Carbohydrates:	*50%*
Fat:	*16%*

MAIN DISH
Crab Loaf with Creamed Peas*🄵

These leftovers make great sandwiches.

Vegetable cooking spray
½ cup fresh rice bread crumbs
¼ cup nonfat Lactaid milk
½ teaspoon sage
2 egg whites, lightly beaten
1 pound canned crabmeat,
   drained

¼ teaspoon salt
½ teaspoon onion powder
1 jar (7½ ounces) junior
   creamed peas baby food,
   warmed

Preheat oven to 350°F. Coat 8"×4"×3" loaf pan with cooking spray. In medium bowl, combine all ingredients except peas. Lightly pack into loaf pan. Bake 45 minutes or until table knife inserted in center comes out clean. Let stand 5 minutes. Turn out onto serving platter and spoon peas down center.

Makes 4 servings

Calories:	*140*
Protein:	*56%*
Carbohydrates:	*26%*
Fat:	*18%*

*Excellent source of heart-healthy omega–3 fatty acids.

91

Deralee Scanlon, R.D.

MAIN DISH
Chicken Dijon with Fettucine*⒡

This dish tastes so rich it's hard to believe there is no added fat.

2 whole (2 pounds) chicken
 breasts, split
Vegetable cooking spray
3½ cups (8 ounces) sliced
 mushrooms
¼ teaspoon garlic powder
¼ cup dry white wine

¼ cup low-sodium chicken
 broth, defatted
8 ounces fettucine, cooked
1 cup plain low-fat yogurt
2 tablespoons prepared Dijon-
 style mustard (optional)

Bone and skin chicken. Trim excess fat. Coat large skillet with cooking spray. Over medium-high heat, brown chicken in skillet. Add mushrooms, garlic powder, wine, and broth. Reduce heat, cover, and simmer until chicken is cooked, about 30 minutes. Place fettucine on heated serving platter and arrange chicken on top; keep warm. Combine yogurt and mustard and blend into mushroom-broth mixture. Heat, do not boil. Spoon over chicken.

Makes 4 servings

Hints: Health-food stores carry pasta made from American (Jerusalem) Artichokes, if desired.

*Contains wheat.

Calories: 319
Protein: 48%
Carbohydrates: 35%
Fat: 17%

MAIN DISH
Tropical Turkey Breast[F]

When it's cold out you can bring flavors of the tropics home with this easy dish.

1 (2¾ pounds) turkey breast, skinned
¼ cup mango nectar
2 tablespoons honey
1 teaspoon prepared Dijon-style mustard (optional)

¼ teaspoon ginger
¼ teaspoon garlic powder
½ teaspoon onion powder

Place foil on bottom of grill to catch drippings. Surround foil with coals. When coals are ready, place turkey on rack. Cover barbecue and cook 1½ to 2 hours until meat thermometer registers 170°F or juices run clear. In small saucepan, melt margarine. Add remaining ingredients and brush turkey frequently during last 30 minutes. Slice and serve on heated platter.

Makes 8 servings

Hints: Add coals during cooking as needed to maintain heat.

Calories:	202
Protein:	65%
Carbohydrates:	13%
Fat:	22%

MAIN DISH
Hunter's - Style Chicken^F

No one will guess this delicious, one-dish meal was cooked in a snap.

1 (1 pound) whole chicken breast, split
¼ cup cornstarch
½ teaspoon onion powder
½ teaspoon salt
Vegetable cooking spray
3½ cups (8 ounces) sliced mushrooms
4 (12 ounces) medium patty-pan squash, peeled and cut into eighths

¾ cup dry white wine or low-sodium chicken broth, defatted
1 teaspoon tarragon leaves
½ teaspoon thyme leaves
3 (12 ounces) small tomatoes, peeled, seeded, and cut into eighths
2 cups cooked rice, hot

Bone and skin chicken. Trim excess fat. Cut into 1-inch strips. Combine cornstarch, onion powder, and salt in plastic bag. Place chicken in bag and shake to coat lightly. Coat heavy 10-inch skillet with cooking spray. Brown chicken over medium-high heat 1 to 2 minutes. Add mushrooms, squash, wine, and seasonings. Bring to a boil, reduce heat, cover, and simmer 10 minutes until squash is tender. Add tomatoes and simmer 2 minutes until lightly cooked. Spoon over rice.

Makes 4 servings

Calories:	251
Protein:	32%
Carbohydrates:	54%
Fat:	14%

MAIN DISH
Crazy Chinese Lasagna [F]

Of course, the Italians invented lasagna; but this is awfully good, anyway.

Vegetable cooking spray
1 can (28 ounces) peeled and chopped tomatoes
1 can (15 ounces) tomato sauce
¼ cup rice wine or sweet vermouth (optional)
1 teaspoon sesame oil (optional)
1½ cup (3½ ounces) sliced mushrooms
¼ teaspoon garlic powder
½ teaspoon onion powder
½ teaspoon ground fennel
1 tablespoon sweet basil
2 teaspoons oregano
½ teaspoon marjoram
3 bay leaves
½ package (3½ ounces) rice stick noodles
1 package (1 pound) medium tofu, drained and crumbled or 8 ounces low-fat cottage cheese

Preheat oven to 350°F. Coat 12″ × 8″ × 2″ baking dish with cooking spray. In large saucepan, combine tomatoes, tomato sauce, wine, oil, mushrooms, and seasonings. Bring to a boil, reduce heat, cover and simmer 20 minutes. Discard bay leaves. In 5-quart Dutch oven, cook noodles in boiling water according to package directions; drain and set aside. Cover bottom of baking dish with 2 cups sauce. Top with layer of half noodles, half tofu and 2 cups sauce. Repeat layers, ending with sauce. Bake 45 minutes.

Makes 6 to 8 servings

Hints: Sesame oil and rice stick noodles can be found in the Oriental or ethnic section of most supermarkets.

Calories:	175
Protein:	18%
Carbohydrates:	56%
Fat:	26%

MAIN DISH
Herbed Fish and Tomato Stew[F]

The convenience of frozen fish fillets means the ingredients can be kept on hand for an easy, hearty meal anytime.

½ teaspoon onion powder
¼ teaspoon garlic powder
1 bay leaf
½ teaspoon thyme
1 bottle (8 ounces) clam juice
¼ cup dry red wine
1 can (28 ounces) peeled and chopped tomatoes
1 (4 ounces) small zucchini, peeled and sliced
2 packages (10 ounces each) frozen cod fillets, quartered
½ lemon, thinly sliced for garnish (optional)

In 5-quart Dutch oven, combine all ingredients except fish and lemon. Bring to a boil, reduce heat, cover, and simmer 15 minutes. Add fish and simmer 5 minutes until fish flakes easily with fork. Garnish with lemon if desired.

Makes 4 servings

Calories:	*167*
Protein:	*67%*
Carbohydrates	*26%*
Fat:	*7%*

MAIN DISH
Crispy Oven-Fried Chicken^F

Seasoned cornmeal gives this no-fuss dish its deliciously crunchy coating.

Vegetable cooking spray
1 (2½ to 3 pounds) broiler-
 fryer chicken, cut up
¾ cup cornmeal

1½ teaspoons dill weed
½ teaspoon salt
½ teaspoon onion powder
¼ teaspoon garlic powder

Preheat oven to 375°F. Coat a 13″ × 9″ × 2″ baking dish with cooking spray. Skin chicken and trim excess fat. In plastic bag, combine cornmeal and seasonings. Dip chicken in water, shaking off excess. Place chicken 2 or 3 pieces at a time in bag and shake to coat. Arrange chicken in baking dish. Bake 30 minutes. Turn chicken over and bake 20 minutes longer or until chicken is golden brown and tender.

Makes 6 servings

Calories:	*270*
Protein:	*52%*
Carbohydrates:	*18%*
Fat:	*30%*

MAIN DISH
Oat and Herb Baked Chicken[F]

This flavorful chicken always wins rave reviews.

Vegetable cooking spray
½ cup oat flour
½ teaspoon paprika
1 teaspoon poultry seasoning

1½ pounds chicken breast
    fillets, about 6 halves
2 tablespoons ketchup
2 tablespoons applesauce

Preheat oven to 375°F. Coat 12″ × 9″ × 2″ baking dish with cooking spray. In plastic bag, combine flour and seasonings. Discard skin and trim excess fat. Place half of chicken at a time in seasoned flour and shake to coat. Place chicken in baking dish. Bake 45 minutes until chicken is browned and tender. Combine ketchup and applesauce and spread on chicken. Bake 5 minutes longer.

Makes 4 servings

Calories:	267
Protein:	65%
Carbohydrates:	16%
Fat:	19%

MAIN DISH
Turkey Meat Loaf^F

Enjoy turkey year round. Ground turkey is now available in most markets fresh and frozen, but it is ground with the skin included. For this recipe, in order to sharply reduce fat content, you must buy turkey breast and have the butcher remove the skin before grinding for you.

Vegetable cooking spray
2 pounds turkey breast
  (without skin), ground
1 cup stale rice bread cubes,
  about 1 slice
1 (5 ounces) Granny Smith
  apple, cored, peeled, and
  chopped

½ teaspoon onion powder
½ teaspoon poultry seasoning
1 egg white, lightly beaten
⅓ cup water
1 jar (4½ ounces) applesauce
  and cherries baby food

Preheat oven to 350°F. Coat 9" × 5" × 3" loaf pan with cooking spray. In large bowl, lightly combine ground turkey, bread, and apple. Mix in seasonings, egg white, and water. Lightly pack into loaf pan. Bake 1 hour. Remove from oven, drain pan juice and let cool 10 minutes before slicing. Garnish with applesauce.

Makes 8 servings

Hints: Leftovers make great sandwiches.

Calories:	*210*
Protein:	*66%*
Carbohydrates:	*18%*
Fat:	*16%*

MAIN DISH
Turkey Pot Roast[F]

Turkey time can be anytime. Try this new twist on two American favorites.

Vegetable cooking spray
1 (2¾ pounds) turkey breast
2¾ cups water, divided
½ teaspoon onion powder
¼ teaspoon garlic powder
½ teaspoon sweet basil
¼ teaspoon thyme
3 (1¼ pounds) medium potatoes, peeled and quartered
4 (1½ pounds) carrots, cut into chunks
1 (10 ounces) sweet potato, peeled and cut into chunks
2 tablespoons cornstarch

Preheat oven to 450°F. Coat 5-quart Dutch oven with cooking spray. Add turkey and 1 cup water; bake 25 minutes until skin crisps. Drain liquid, reserving broth. Discard fat and turkey skin. Return broth and turkey to pan. Add seasonings, vegetables, and 1½ cups water. Reduce heat to 350°F. Cover and bake 45 minutes until vegetables are tender. Remove turkey and vegetables to heated platter; keep warm. Dissolve cornstarch in ¼ cup water and stir into pan juices. Bring to a boil, stirring constantly.

Makes 4 servings

Hints: For more flavorful gravy, add ¼ cup dry red wine before thickening.

Calories:	*305*
Protein:	*63%*
Carbohydrates:	*20%*
Fat:	*17%*

MAIN DISH
Shrimp 'n' Rice Casserole[F]

An easy, healthy dish for buffet or busy-day dining.

2 cans (10½ ounces each) low-sodium chicken broth, defatted
1 cup brown rice
¼ cup dry sherry (optional)
1 cup (3 ounces) sliced mushrooms

½ teaspoon onion powder
1 pound small cooked shrimp
1 teaspoon dill weed
3 egg whites, lightly beaten
Vegetable cooking spray

In medium saucepan, bring broth to a boil and add rice and sherry. Reduce heat, cover, and simmer 25 minutes. Add mushrooms and onion powder and simmer 5 minutes longer. Remove from heat and add shrimp and dill. Whisk in eggs. Preheat oven to 350°F. Coat 2-quart casserole with cooking spray. Spoon mixture into casserole. Bake 50 minutes. Let stand 10 minutes.

Makes 4 servings

Hints: As baked casserole stands, excess moisture will be absorbed.

Calories:	*332*
Protein:	*36%*
Carbohydrates:	*56%*
Fat:	*8%*

SOUP

Pumpkin- Apple Cream Soup^F

The flavors of pumpkin and apple are a harmonious blend in this thick cream soup.

2 tablespoons margarine
1 small (¾ cup) finely
   chopped, peeled baking
   apple
1 tablespoon potato starch
2 cans (14½ ounces each)
   defatted, low-sodium
   chicken broth

1 can (1 pound 13 ounces)
   pumpkin
¼ teaspoon maple flavoring
1 cup low-fat Lactaid milk
Plain low-fat yogurt for
   garnish
Apple slices for garnish

In 5-quart Dutch oven, melt margarine; sauté apple until transparent. Stir in starch, mixing well. Gradually add broth, stirring constantly. Add pumpkin and maple extract. Cook over low heat, stirring constantly until mixture boils. Gradually add milk, stirring constantly. Heat thoroughly. To serve, place dollop of yogurt and apple slice on each small bowl of soup.

Makes about 7 cups

Hints: If soup thickens, add more milk. If desired (and if you can tolerate them) add ½ teaspoon nutmeg and ½ teaspoon cinnamon to soup before simmering.
In the fall, serve soup in mini-pumpkins, cleaned, with seeds and fibers removed. Then use the pumpkins as a container for bread stuffing; bake the pumpkins in 350°F. oven about 1 hour or until pumpkin is softened.

Deralee Scanlon, R.D.

Calories:	106
Protein:	11%
Carbohydrates:	64%
Fat:	25%

SOUP
Lee Chou's Egg Drop Soup^[F]

Who says you're hungry in an hour . . . not with this soup.

2 cans (10½ ounces each) low-sodium chicken broth, defatted
1 can water
¼ cup brown rice
2 stalks celery, halved
1 (6 ounces) large carrot, diagonally sliced
¼ teaspoon thyme
1 (1 pound) whole chicken breast, split, skin removed and boned

½ package (5 ounces) frozen chopped spinach, thawed and drained
1 tablespoon lemon juice
1 egg, beaten
1 teaspoon sesame oil
1 tablespoon cornstarch
¼ cup water

In 5-quart Dutch oven, combine broth, water, rice, celery, carrot, and thyme. Bring to a boil, reduce heat, cover, and simmer 30 minutes. Cut chicken into 2" × ⅓" × ⅓" slivers. Add chicken, return to a boil, and simmer 3 minutes. Discard celery. Add spinach and juice, return to a boil, and simmer 5 minutes. Pour egg in thin stream into soup, stirring constantly. Add oil. Dissolve cornstarch in water and stir into soup; return to a boil, stirring constantly. Serve in heated soup bowls.

Makes 4 servings

Hints: For a meatless entrée or soup course, omit chicken.

Calories: 221
Protein: 34%
Carbohydrates: 37%
Fat: 29%

SOUP
Halibut Chowder[F]

A feast on a cool evening.

1 bottle (8 ounces) clam juice
1 quart water
6 (1¾ pounds) small russet
  potatoes, peeled and
  quartered
¼ teaspoon onion powder
¼ teaspoon thyme
½ teaspoon salt

½ teaspoon dill weed
1½ pounds halibut, skin
  removed and cut into 1-inch
  cubes
⅓ cup plain nonfat yogurt
Fresh dill sprigs for garnish
  (optional)

In 5-quart Dutch oven, combine clam juice, water, potatoes, and seasonings. Bring to a boil, reduce heat, cover and simmer 20 minutes until potatoes are tender. With slotted spoon, remove potatoes to blender or food processor. Add small amount of cooking liquid and purée until smooth. Return potato mixture to pan. Add halibut and cook 5 minutes until it flakes easily with fork. Remove from heat and stir in yogurt. Spoon into warm soup bowls. Garnish with dill sprig if desired.

Makes 6 servings

Calories:	161
Protein:	65%
Carbohydrates:	28%
Fat*:	7%

*Excellent source of heart-healthy omega-3 fatty acids.

SOUP
Vegetable- Millet Soup^F

Steaming hot, this soup is satisfying, colorful, and just right for lunch or dinner.

¼ cup millet
3 cups low-sodium chicken broth or water
¼ cup dry sherry (optional)
½ teaspoon garlic powder
½ teaspoon salt
1 stalk celery, halved
1 (5 ounces) small Japanese eggplant, peeled and cubed

½ pound small mushrooms
2 (6 ounces) small patty-pan squash, peeled and sliced
1 (5 ounces) medium tomato; peeled, seeded, and quartered

In 5-quart Dutch oven, combine millet, broth, sherry, garlic powder, salt, and celery. Bring to a boil, reduce heat, cover, and simmer 45 minutes. Discard celery. Add eggplant and simmer 10 minutes. Add remaining vegetables and simmer 15 minutes longer. Serve in heated soup bowls.

Makes 4 servings

Hints: Millet is available in health-food stores.

Calories:	*130*
Protein:	*16%*
Carbohydrates:	*70%*
Fat:	*14%*

DESSERT
Meringued Poached Pears

A dessert that is sure to be a hit . . . for family or guests.

1½ cups water
2 tablespoons honey
1 teaspoon vanilla extract

4 to 6 firm pears; peeled,
cored, and halved

Topping:

2 tablespoons margarine
2 tablespoons packed brown
sugar

2 tablespoons wheat germ
(optional)

Meringue:

3 egg whites
Pinch salt
Pinch cream of tartar

¼ cup granulated sugar
¼ teaspoon vanilla extract

In medium saucepan, combine water, honey, and vanilla. Bring to a boil, stirring until sugar is dissolved. Gently add pears. Cover and simmer 10 to 15 minutes (depending upon type and size of pears) or until tender. Remove from pan; cover and chill in syrup 2 to 4 hours.

Topping: In small saucepan, melt margarine. Add sugar. Stir over low heat until sugar is dissolved. Add wheat germ. Set aside. Mixture will harden slightly; crumble before adding to pears.

Meringue: In medium glass or metal bowl, beat egg whites until foamy. Beat in salt and cream of tartar. Continue beating until soft peaks form. Gradually add sugar, beating until stiff peaks form. Blend in vanilla.

Preheat oven to 425°F. In 10″ baking dish, arrange well-drained pears. Spoon meringue in center, mounding it in middle. Sprinkle brown sugar mixture around edges. Bake 4 to 5 minutes or until meringue is lightly browned. Serve immediately.

Makes 8 to 12 servings (one-half pear per serving)

Calories:	109
Protein:	3%
Carbohydrates:	80%
Fat:	17%

DESSERT
Maple Apple Crisp

Serve this sugar 'n' spice dessert warm.

Vegetable cooking spray
4 cups thinly sliced, peeled
  Granny Smith apples
2 tablespoons water
1 tablespoon lemon juice
3 tablespoons maple syrup

½ cup quick oats, uncooked
3 tablespoons packed dark
  brown sugar
3 tablespoons margarine,
  melted
Plain low-fat yogurt (optional)

Preheat oven to 375°F. Coat 8″ × 8″ × 2″ baking dish with cooking spray. In large bowl, combine apples, water, juice, and syrup. Arrange mixture in baking dish. In small bowl, combine oats, brown sugar, and margarine, and crumble over apple mixture. Bake 30 minutes or until fruit is tender and topping is crisp. Serve immediately with dollop of yogurt if desired.

Makes 6 servings

Calories:	169
Protein:	2%
Carbohydrates:	68%
Fat:	30%

DESSERT
Light Peach Cobbler*

Surprisingly light and definitely delicious.

Vegetable cooking spray
2 cans (16 ounces each) sliced
  peaches in light syrup
3 tablespoons quick-cooking
  tapioca
2 tablespoons maple syrup
¼ cup oat flour
¼ cup all-purpose flour
1 tablespoon granulated sugar

1 teaspoon baking powder
Pinch cardamom
1 egg, lightly beaten
2 tablespoons low-fat Lactaid
  milk
2 tablespoons vegetable oil
1 teaspoon granulated sugar
  (optional)

Preheat oven to 400°F. Coat 1-quart casserole with cooking spray. Drain peaches, reserving 1¼ cups syrup. In small saucepan, combine syrup, tapioca, and maple syrup. Bring to a boil, reduce heat, and simmer 1 minute, stirring constantly. Place peaches and syrup in casserole. In small bowl, combine flours, 1 tablespoon sugar, baking powder, and cardamom. Stir in egg, milk, and oil; do not overmix. Drop 12 small teaspoons of mixture onto fruit. Sprinkle with 1 tablespoon sugar if desired. Bake 25 minutes or until golden brown.

Makes 8 servings

Calories:	167
Protein:	4%
Carbohydrates:	74%
Fat:	22%

*Contains wheat.

DESSERT
Grandma's Rice Pudding

Definitely a comfort food.

1 cup low-fat Lactaid milk
1 cup cooked rice
¼ cup granulated sugar
1 tablespoon oat flour

Pinch salt
1 egg, lightly beaten
1 teaspoon vanilla extract
Vegetable cooking spray

In heavy saucepan, scald milk, stirring frequently. Add rice. Combine sugar, flour, and salt. Whisk into milk mixture. Bring to a boil, reduce heat, and simmer, stirring constantly for 5 minutes or until thickened. Stir small amount of hot mixture into egg. Then whisk egg back into hot mixture. Add vanilla. Coat 1½-quart baking dish with cooking spray. Bake in 300°F oven for 30 minutes or until knife inserted in center comes out clean. Serve warm.

Makes 6 servings

Calories:	*105*
Protein:	*11%*
Carbohydrates:	*72%*
Fat:	*17%*

DESSERT
Old-Fashioned Bundt Cake*Ⓕ

This recipe will be such a favorite it will disappear from the cake plate.

Vegetable cooking spray
¾ cup vegetable oil
1 cup granulated sugar
½ cup honey
1 teaspoon vanilla extract
2 eggs
3⅓ cups cake flour

½ teaspoon ground cardamom
2 teaspoons baking soda
¼ teaspoon salt
1 cup buttermilk
2 tablespoons powdered
  sugar, sifted

Preheat oven to 350°F. Coat large bundt pan or fluted mold with cooking spray. In large bowl, beat oil, granulated sugar, and honey until fluffy. Beat in vanilla and eggs. Combine flour, cardamom, soda, and salt; beat into egg mixture, alternating with buttermilk, until smooth. Bake for 1½ hours or until toothpick inserted in center comes out clean. Let cool on rack 10 minutes. Turn cake out onto rack to cool completely. Dust with powdered sugar.

Makes 12 to 15 servings

Note: This cake is high in calories per serving. While it is not used in any of the following menu plans for that reason, you may wish to enjoy it as part of a festive occasion when it is difficult to find a "safe" special dessert.

*Contains wheat

Calories: 273
Protein: 6%
Carbohydrates: 67%
Fat: 27%

DESSERT
Indian Pudding[F]

A traditional Early American dessert.

Vegetable cooking spray
3 cups low-fat Lactaid milk
½ cup cornmeal
½ teaspoon maple flavoring
⅓ cup honey

1 egg
¼ teaspoon ginger
Pinch salt
1 (5 ounces) apple; cored,
   peeled, and chopped

Preheat oven to 300°F. Coat 1½-quart casserole with cooking spray. In top of double boiler over hot water, heat milk. Whisk cornmeal into milk and cook until mixture thickens. Combine flavoring, honey, egg, ginger, and salt; whisk into cornmeal mixture. Stir in chopped apple. Pour into casserole. Cover and bake 1½ hours. Serve hot.

Makes 6 to 8 servings

Calories:	171
Protein:	14%
Carbohydrates:	65%
Fat:	21%

BREADS
Rice Spoon Bread

Remember corn spoon bread? This is a version using cream of rice cereal.

Vegetable cooking spray
2 cups water
1 teaspoon vegetable oil
½ cup quick cream of rice
  cereal
1 jar (4½ ounces) strained
  creamed corn baby food

¾ cup nonfat Lactaid milk
½ teaspoon dill weed
½ teaspoon onion powder
2 egg whites

Preheat oven to 350°F. Coat 2-quart soufflé dish with cooking spray. In top of double boiler, bring water and oil to a boil. Gradually whisk in cream of rice. Place over hot water and cook 20 to 30 minutes until all water is absorbed, stirring occasionally. Add creamed corn, milk, and seasonings. In medium glass or metal bowl, beat egg whites until soft peaks form. Gently fold into rice mixture so as not to reduce volume. Pour into soufflé dish and bake 35 to 45 minutes until lightly browned. Serve immediately.

Makes 6 servings

Hints: Serve this in place of a starch at dinner.

Calories:	*45*
Protein:	*21%*
Carbohydrates:	*61%*
Fat:	*18%*

BREADS
Zucchini-Carrot Bread*□

Flavorful and moist. A "must" for healthy snacking.

Vegetable cooking spray
3 egg whites
¼ cup honey
¼ cup packed golden brown
   sugar
1½ teaspoons maple flavoring

½ cup shredded zucchini
½ cup shredded carrots
1¼ cups all-purpose flour
1 teaspoon baking soda
¼ teaspoon salt
3 tablespoons vegetable oil

Preheat oven to 350°F. Coat 9″×5″×3″ loaf pan with cooking spray. In large bowl, beat egg whites. Add honey, sugar, and flavoring. Stir in zucchini and carrot. Combine flour, baking soda, and salt. Stir into zucchini mixture alternating with oil; do not overmix. Spread batter in loaf pan. Bake 50 to 60 minutes or until toothpick inserted in center comes out clean. Cool in pan 10 minutes; turn out onto rack to cool completely.

Makes 1 loaf (12 servings)

Calories:	117
Protein:	7%
Carbohydrates:	66%
Fat:	27%

*Contains wheat.

BREADS
Skillet Corn Bread*☐

This hearty corn bread is a perfect accompaniment to soups and main dish salads.

Vegetable cooking spray
1 cup all-purpose flour
1 cup cornmeal
¾ cup instant potato flakes
1 tablespoon baking powder
¼ teaspoon salt
1 tablespoon granulated sugar
3½ teaspoons margarine,
   melted

4 egg whites, slightly beaten
1 jar (4½ ounce) creamed corn
   baby food
1¼ cups nonfat Lactaid milk
¼ cup quick oats, uncooked

Preheat oven to 400°F. Coat 10″ skillet with cooking spray. In large bowl, combine flour, cornmeal, potato flakes, baking powder, salt, and sugar. Stir in margarine, egg whites, corn, and milk; do not overmix. Spread batter in skillet. Sprinkle with oats. Bake 30 to 35 minutes or until toothpick inserted in center comes out clean. Cut into wedges.

Makes 12 servings, each approximately a 3″ wedge

Calories:	210
Protein:	12%
Carbohydrates:	58%
Fat:	30%

*Contains wheat

BREADS
Cornmeal Scones*F

A nice pick-me-up with tea in the afternoon . . . hearty when served with soup.

⅓ cup potato starch
⅔ cup all-purpose flour
½ cup cornmeal
¼ cup granulated sugar
1 tablespoon baking powder

¼ teaspoon salt
⅔ cup nonfat Lactaid milk
3½ tablespoons margarine, melted

Preheat oven to 375°F. In medium bowl, combine starch, flour, cornmeal, sugar, baking powder, and salt. Stir in milk and margarine; do not overmix. On waxed paper, pat out dough to 8″ square. Freeze 15 minutes until slightly firm. Cut into quarters to form four 4″ squares; cut each square diagonally into quarters to form 16 triangles. Separate triangles and place on ungreased cookie sheet. Bake 20 minutes. Serve warm with honey or jam.

Makes 16 scones

Hints: Dough will seem too wet while you are working with it; it cuts easily after being in the freezer.

Calories:	78
Protein:	5%
Carbohydrates:	65%
Fat:	30%

*Contains wheat.

BREADS
Honey-Oat Muffins *F

Pop some of these in the freezer for later.

Vegetable cooking spray
3 tablespoons vegetable oil
⅓ cup honey
3 tablespoons granulated
   sugar
1 egg

1 cup all-purpose flour
1¼ cups oat flour
1 tablespoon baking powder
¼ teaspoon salt
¾ cup low-fat Lactaid milk

Preheat oven to 425°F. Coat muffin cups with cooking spray or line with paper baking cups. In large bowl, beat oil, honey, and sugar until creamed. Beat in egg. Combine flours, baking powder, and salt; stir into egg mixture, alternating with milk until combined. Do not overmix. Spoon batter into muffin cups. Bake 16 to 18 minutes or until toothpick inserted in center comes out clean.

Makes 1 dozen

Calories:	147
Protein:	8%
Carbohydrates:	62%
Fat:	30%

*Contains wheat.

SIDE DISH
Potato - Mushroom Bake[F]

Prepare this early in the day, then just bake before serving.

Vegetable cooking spray
3 (1 pound) small potatoes, peeled and sliced
2 cups (6 ounces) sliced mushrooms
½ teaspoon onion powder

½ teaspoon salt
1 teaspoon tarragon leaves
1 cup low-fat Lactaid milk

Preheat oven to 350°F. Coat 10″ × 6″ × 2″ baking dish with cooking spray. Layer half potatoes and half mushrooms, seasoning each layer with mixture of onion powder, salt, and tarragon. Repeat layers. Pour milk over top. Cover with foil and bake 45 minutes. Remove foil and bake 30 minutes longer or until potatoes are tender.

Makes 6 servings

Calories:	77
Protein:	21%
Carbohydrates:	67%
Fat:	12%

SIDE DISH
Summer Garden Stir-Fry

We've combined our garden bounty of fruit and vegetables in an unusual and delicious way.

1 teaspoon olive oil
1 (8 ounces) large Japanese
  eggplant, peeled and diced
1 (4 ounces) small zucchini,
  sliced diagonally
1 (4 ounces) small tomato;
  peeled, seeded, and diced

1 (6 ounces) nectarine, peeled
  and thinly sliced
2 teaspoons minced dried
  basil, or fresh if tolerated

In large skillet over medium-high heat, heat oil. Stir-fry eggplant and zucchini 15 minutes until tender. Add tomato and nectarine. Reduce heat, cover, and simmer 10 minutes. Sprinkle with basil before serving.

Makes 4 servings

Calories:	54
Protein:	7%
Carbohydrates:	74%
Fat:	19%

SIDE DISH
Brown Rice Salad Vinaigrette

The freshness of mint flavors this delightfully refreshing salad.

2 cups water
1 cup brown rice
2 tablespoons rice vinegar
1 teaspoon dried mint leaves, crushed
2 teaspoons extra-light olive oil

Romaine lettuce leaves for garnish
2 (8 ounces) nectarines, peeled and sliced

In medium saucepan, bring water to a boil. Add rice, stir, and cover. Bring to a boil, reduce heat, and simmer about 45 minutes or until rice is tender. Remove from heat and let stand 5 minutes. Combine vinegar and mint; blend. Gradually add olive oil, beating well. Pour over hot rice. Let stand at room temperature at least 1 hour before serving or chill 2 to 3 hours in refrigerator. If refrigerated, let stand 1 hour at room temperature before serving. To serve, arrange lettuce leaves in shallow serving bowl. Mound rice in center. Arrange nectarine slices around rice.

Makes 4 servings

Calories:	90
Protein:	5%
Carbohydrates:	68%
Fat:	27%

SIDE DISH
Sweet Pilaf

This side dish complements both fish and chicken.

1¼ cups apple juice or low-
   sodium chicken broth
½ cup brown rice
¼ cup dry sherry (optional)

¼ teaspoon salt
1 tablespoon margarine
1 (3 ounces) carrot, sliced
1 medium peach

In medium saucepan, bring juice to a boil. Add rice, sherry, salt, margarine, and carrot. Reduce heat, cover, and simmer 35 minutes. Add peach and simmer 10 minutes longer.

Makes 4 servings

Calories:	*156*
Protein:	*5%*
Carbohydrates:	*78%*
Fat:	*17%*

SIDE DISH
Roasted Rosemary Potatoes[F]

Quick and easy. Good served with any main dish . . . or even snacking.

Vegetable cooking spray
4 small (1¼ pounds) russet
  potatoes

½ to 1 teaspoon rosemary,
  crushed
½ teaspoon onion powder

Preheat oven to 450°F. Coat shallow baking pan lightly with cooking spray. Cut each potato lengthwise into 8 wedges. Place cut side up in baking pan. Coat lightly with cooking spray. Sprinkle with rosemary and onion powder. Bake 20 minutes until tender.

Makes 4 servings

Calories:	57
Protein:	10%
Carbohydrates:	90%
Fat:	0%

SIDE DISH
Oriental Oat Pilaf

A flavorful side dish to serve with fish or chicken.

1 cup quick oats, uncooked
1 egg white, lightly beaten
1 cup oyster or small button
   mushrooms
½ cup peeled, seeded, and
   diced cucumber
1½ teaspoons margarine
¾ to 1 cup low-sodium
   chicken broth, defatted

½ teaspoon sesame oil
1 teaspoon granulated sugar
2 star anise (optional)
2 ounces tofu, drained, rinsed
   and cubed or ¼ cup low-fat
   cottage cheese

In medium bowl, comine oats and egg white. In medium skillet over medium-high heat, stir-fry mushrooms and cucumber in margarine 3 minutes. Add oat mixture and stir-fry 8 minutes until oats are dry and lightly browned. Add broth, oil, sugar, and star anise. Reduce heat, cover, and simmer 3 to 5 minutes or until liquid is absorbed. Discard star anise. Stir in tofu and heat through.

Makes 4 servings

Hints: Star anise is available in spice stores or Oriental supermarkets. To easily de-fat chicken broth, chill broth then skim fat.

Calories:	*135*
Protein:	*19%*
Carbohydrates:	*53%*
Fat:	*28%*

SIDE DISH
Stuffed Acorn Squash

Whether you are a vegetarian or just enjoy an occasional meatless entrée, this makes a delightful meal.

Vegetable cooking spray
2 (5 pounds) large acorn or butternut squash
3½ cups (8 ounces) sliced mushrooms
2 (12 ounces) delicious apples; cored, peeled, and coarsely chopped

½ teaspoon onion powder
¼ teaspoon garlic powder
1 teaspoon sweet basil
¼ teaspoon sage
1 cup fresh rice bread crumbs
¼ cup low-sodium chicken broth (water may be substituted)

Preheat oven to 350°F. Coat baking sheet with cooking spray. Cut squash in half lengthwise; remove seeds. Place squash cut side down on baking sheet. Bake 1 hour. Meanwhile, prepare the filling. Coat medium skillet with cooking spray. Over medium-high heat, sauté mushrooms, apples, and seasonings 15 minutes. Add crumbs and broth; toss lightly to mix. Fill squash with stuffing. Cover and bake 30 minutes longer until squash is tender.

Makes 4 servings

Hints: To use as a side dish, cut squash pieces in half before serving.

Calories:	156
Protein:	14%
Carbohydrates:	79%
Fat:	7%

SIDE DISH
Rice and Potato Pancakes *ⓕ

Try these for a hearty breakfast with applesauce and plain yogurt or have them at dinner with a light gravy . . . delicious either way.

1 small apple; peeled, cored, and chopped
1 egg
2 cups peeled and cubed potatoes
1 cup cold, cooked brown rice
½ cup low-fat Lactaid milk

2 tablespoons all-purpose flour
1 tablespoon margarine, melted
1 teaspoon granulated sugar
¼ teaspoon salt
Vegetable cooking spray

In food processor fitted with steel blade or blender, purée apple with egg. Add potatoes, one half at a time, and purée. Add rice, milk, flour, margarine, sugar, and salt and process until smooth. Over medium heat, heat griddle or heavy skillet. Heavily coat griddle with cooking spray. Pour ¼ cup batter for each pancake on griddle. Lightly coat top side of pancake with cooking spray before turning. Cook until well browned on each side. Serve immediately.

Makes 10 pancakes

Hints: Pancakes may be prepared ahead and cooled on rack. To reheat, place rack on baking sheet and heat for 15 minutes in 350°F oven.

*Contains wheat.

131

Calories:	79
Protein:	*15%*
Carbohydrates:	*66%*
Fat:	*19%*

SIDE DISH
Glazed Carrots[F]

Always an easy favorite . . . these have a hint of pineapple.

1 cup water
1 can (6 ounces) pineapple
  juice

6 (1 pound) carrots, julienned
1 tablespoon packed dark
  brown sugar

In large saucepan, combine water, juice, and carrots. Bring to a boil, reduce heat, cover, and simmer 15 minutes. Drain reserving liquid. Return liquid to pan. Boil mixture to reduce to ¼ cup. Add sugar. Add carrots and coat with glaze.

Makes 4 servings

Calories:	102
Protein:	8%
Carbohydrates:	92%
Fat:	0%

THIRTY-DAY BASIC
COMFORT MEAL PLANS

I.B.S. is a highly individual ailment: as the saying goes, "One man's food is another man's poison."

However, the daily meal plans on the following pages contain only foods generally considered to be comfortable for most I.B.S. patients during periods of symptoms distress. All of the preceding fifty recipes are used here, while foods on our "avoid" list have been completely omitted.

Each day's meals are balanced to include the basic food groups; the one exception is that milk products have been held off until the second week to help you check for any possible condition of lactose intolerance.

For reasons explained earlier (see page 50), each day has been divided into six reasonably sized meals in order to prevent overeating at any one time. Snacks are recommended for 10 A.M., 3 P.M., and 9 P.M. Try not to skip meals; if you do, you may be overly hungry later and tend to binge.

As an added convenience, every effort has been made to utilize leftovers within an appropriate period of time.

Before you embark on this thirty-day cycle, you may wish to reread pages 60-61 of this book, which further explain the proper and effective use of these Basic Comfort Meal Plans.

MENU PLANS: DAY 1

Breakfast:
307
calories

1 scrambled egg
¼ cup chopped spinach
1 slice whole-wheat toast
1 pat margarine
¾ cup fruit nectar

Snack:
198
calories

1 honey-baked apple (plain baked)
1 English muffin
1 teaspoon jam

Lunch:
395
calories

½ broiled chicken breast
¼ medium baked yam
½ cup steamed, sliced zucchini
1 whole-wheat roll
1 pat margarine

Snack:
200
calories

1 serving Vegetable Millet Soup
2 rice cakes

Dinner:
555
calories

Turkey Meat Loaf
1 cup mashed potatoes
½ cup green peas
1 pat margarine
½ cup fruit cocktail (packed in fruit juice)

Snack:
102
calories

½ cup canned cherries
2 vanilla wafers

Total Daily Calories: 1,757
(Note: Since dairy foods have been omitted for the first week, a calcium supplement may be advisable. The RDA for calcium is 800 mg.)

MENU PLANS: DAY 2

Breakfast:
290
calories

1 ready-to-eat whole-wheat waffle
1 tablespoon maple syrup
4 apricot halves (in fruit juice)

1 pat margarine
1 cup decaffeinated tea

Snack:
180
calories

1 slice toast
1 turkey frankfurter
1 tablespoon ketchup

Lunch:
395
calories

1 serving Lee Chou's Egg
    Drop Soup (freeze)
1 serving cucumber and
    tomato slices (no dressing)
5 Melba Toast
½ cup fruit nectar

Snack:
204
calories

1/12 cake, angel food (freeze)
1 jar strained Dutch apple
    infant fruit

Dinner:
585
calories

1 serving Crispy Oven-Fried
    Chicken
1 small baked potato
1 pat margarine
1 cup chopped spinach
1 cup stewed eggplant and
    tomatoes
2 canned pineapple rings
    (packed in juice)

Snack:
94
calories

½ cup fruit cocktail
2 ginger snaps

Total Daily Calories: 1,748

MENU PLANS: DAY 3

Breakfast:
294
calories

1 poached egg
1 bagel
1 pat margarine

½ cup diluted grapefruit
juice (50/50 with water)

Snack:
176
calories

1 slice toast
1 pat margarine
1 tablespoon jelly

Lunch:
377
calories

1 Turkey Meat Loaf
Sandwich with mustard
on 2 slices whole-wheat
bread
1 slice tomato
1 dill pickle
1 cup decaffeinated tea or
spring water

Snack:
200
calories

1 serving Vegetable Millet
Soup
2 rice cakes

Dinner:
596
calories

4 ounces Lemon-Broiled
Swordfish
1 serving Roasted Rosemary
Potatoes
1 pat margarine
1 cup steamed green peas
and crookneck squash
1 serving Maple Apple Crisp

Snack:
102
calories

½ cup canned cherries
2 vanilla wafers

Total Daily Calories: 1,745

MENU PLANS: DAY 4

Breakfast:
279
calories

¾ cup cooked cereal
½ English muffin
1 pat margarine
2 teaspoons sugar or honey
1 cup decaffeinated tea

Snack:
185
calories

1 toasted bagel
1 tablespoon jelly

Lunch:
409
calories

1 serving Chicken Squash-
Rice Soup
1 whole wheat roll
1 pat butter
5 stewed plums

Snack:
194
calories

½ cup vegetable juice
1 serving Maple Apple Crisp

Dinner:
562
calories

½ cup fruit nectar
1 serving Tropical Turkey
Breast
1 serving brown rice
vinaigrette salad
½ cup sliced, steamed beets
1 whole-wheat dinner roll
1 pat margarine
1 small peeled pear

Snack:
114
calories

2 canned peach halves
(packed in juice)
2 graham crackers

Total Daily Calories: 1,743

MENU PLANS: DAY 5

Breakfast:
309 calories

1 fried egg
1 slice whole-wheat toast
1 pat margarine (unless some has been used to fry egg)
1 tablespoon jam
½ cup canned cherries (no pits)

Snack:
198 calories

1 plain baked apple
1 English muffin
1 teaspoon jam

Lunch:
398 calories

1 serving Vegetable Millet Soup
3-ounce scoop of tuna
2 teaspoons mayonnaise
2 rice cakes
½ cup vegetable juice

Snack:
208 calories

1 serving Chicken Squash Rice Soup
1 Saltine cracker

Dinner:
597 calories

1 serving Oat Herb-Baked Chicken
1 cup stewed tomatoes and French-cut green beans
½ medium sweet potato
½ cup fruit nectar
½ cup applesauce

Snack:
94 calories

½ cup fruit cocktail (packed in juice)
2 ginger snaps

Total Daily Calories: 1,804

MENU PLANS: DAY 6

Breakfast:
293
calories

¾ cup cooked cereal
½ bagel
1 pat margarine
¼ cup applesauce
1 teaspoon jelly

Snack:
185
calories

1 toasted bagel
1 tablespoon jelly

Lunch:
377
calories

1 Turkey Meat Loaf
    Sandwich with mustard
    on 2 slices whole-wheat
    bread
1 slice tomato
1 dill pickle
1 cup decaffeinated tea or
    spring water

Snack:
190
calories

1 medium baked potato with
    creamed spinach
1 pat margarine

Dinner:
610
calories

½ cup fruit nectar
1 serving Broiled Fillet of
    Sole with lemon wedge
1 cup brown rice
½ cup crookneck squash
1 plain baked apple
1 pat margarine

Snack:
114
calories

2 canned peach halves
    (packed in juice)
2 graham crackers

Total Daily Calories: 1,769

MENU PLANS: DAY 7

Breakfast:
305
calories

1 ready-to-eat whole-wheat waffle
1 tablespoon jelly
1 nectarine
1 cup diluted grapefruit juice (50/50 with water)

Snack:
176
calories

1 slice toast
1 pat margarine
1 tablespoon sugar
1 cup decaffeinated tea

Lunch:
398
calories

1 serving Chicken Squash-Rice Soup
6 Saltine crackers
2 canned peach halves (packed in juice)
½ cup fruit nectar

Snack:
200 calories

1 serving Vegetable Millet Soup
2 rice cakes

Dinner:
607
calories

1 serving Tropical Turkey Breast
1 cup brown rice
1 pat margarine
¾ cup banana squash
1 cup canned fruit cocktail (packed in juice)

Snack:
102
calories

2 canned pear halves (packed in juice)
2 vanilla wafers

Total Daily Calories: 1,788

MENU PLANS: DAY 8

Breakfast:
374
calories

1 poached egg
1 toasted English muffin
1 cup nonfat Lactaid milk
1 pat butter or 1 teaspoon jam

Snack:
192
calories

1 honey-oat muffin
1 pat margarine

Lunch:
231
calories

Halibut Chowder (freeze)
2 rice cakes
1 cup decaffeinated tea

Snack:
197
calories

4 graham crackers
1 cup nonfat Lactaid milk

Dinner:
590
calories

Lemon Herb Turkey with Brown Rice
1 serving glazed carrots
1 serving meringued poached pears
½ cup vegetable juice
1 honey-baked apple (plain baked with 1 tablespoon honey)

Total Daily Calories: 1,745

MENU PLANS: DAY 9

Breakfast:
293
calories

2 Rice and Potato Pancakes
½ cup plain nonfat yogurt
¾ cup unsweetened applesauce

	1 cup decaffeinated tea or spring water
Snack: 237 calories	1 slice zucchini carrot bread ½ cup fruit nectar
Lunch: 348 calories	3 ounces ground turkey patty (from skinless breast) 1 whole-wheat bun mustard 1 dill pickle 1 teaspoon mayonnaise 1 slice tomato 1 cup decaffeinated tea or spring water
Snack: 200 calories	2 ounces skim mozzarella cheese 4 Saltine crackers
Dinner: 504 calories	Crab Loaf with Creamed Peas 1 serving stuffed acorn squash 2 cornmeal scones 2 pats margarine 1 cup decaffeinated tea
Snack: 195 calories	1 serving Grandma's Rice Pudding 1 cup nonfat Lactaid milk

Total Daily Calories: 1,777

MENU PLANS: DAY 10

Breakfast:
290
calories

¾ cup ready-to-eat cereal
1 cup nonfat Lactaid milk
¾ cup blueberries
½ cup fruit nectar
1 cup decaffeinated tea or
   spring water

Snack:
252
calories

1 honey-oat muffin
1 pat margarine
½ cup fruit nectar

Lunch:
400
calories

Herbed Fish and Tomato
   Stew (freeze)
1 whole-wheat roll
½ cup unsweetened
   applesauce
1 pat margarine
2 steamed patty-pan squash
1 cup decaffeinated tea or
   spring water

Snack:
175
calories

2 graham crackers
1 cup nonfat yogurt
1 tablespoon jam

Dinner:
548
calories

Tarragon Roasted Chicken
   in a Bag
1 serving Potato-Mushroom
   Bake
1 serving Summer Garden
   Stir-Fry
1 serving Vegetable Millet
   Soup
1 cup decaffeinated tea

Snack:
109
calories

1 serving Meringued
Poached Pears

Total Daily Calories: 1,774

MENU PLANS: DAY 11

Breakfast:
312
calories

¾ cup cooked cereal
1 honey-oat muffin
1 pat margarine or 1
   tablespoon jam
1 cup decaffeinated tea or
   spring water

Snack:
195
calories

1 serving Grandma's Rice
   Pudding
1 cup nonfat Lactaid milk

Lunch:
386
calories

Lee Chou's Egg Drop Soup
1 serving cucumber and
   tomato slices
5 melba toast
½ cup pineapple juice

Snack:
187
calories

1 slice Zucchini-Carrot Bread
1 pat margarine
½ cup vegetable juice

Dinner:
583
calories

Scallops à la Maison
1 Cornmeal Scone
1 pat margarine
1 cup steamed green beans
1 serving Meringued
   Poached Pears
½ cup vegetable juice

Snack: 99 calories	2 graham crackers ½ cup nonfat Lactaid milk

Total Daily Calories 1,764

MENU PLANS: DAY 12

Breakfast: 292 calories	1 scrambled egg 1 Cornmeal Scone 1 pat margarine ½ medium cantaloupe 1 cup decaffeinated tea or spring water
Snack: 187 calories	1 slice Zucchini-Carrot Bread 1 pat margarine ½ cup vegetable juice

Lunch:
398
calories
	Toasted cheese sandwich (2
	    ounces skim mozzarella; 2
	    slices whole-wheat bread)
	1 tablespoon mustard
	1 cup vegetable broth
	    bouillon
	½ canned pear (packed in
	    juice)

Snack: 200 calories	6 ginger snaps 1 cup nonfat Lactaid milk
Dinner: 597 calories	Chicken Ratatouille 1 cup brown rice 5 steamed asparagus spears ½ cup sherbet 1 cup decaffeinated tea

Snack:
109
calories

1 serving Meringued
Poached Pears

Total Daily Calories: 1,783

MENU PLANS: DAY 13

Breakfast:
308
calories

1 ready-to-eat whole-wheat
    waffle
½ cup cooked blueberries
½ cup fruit nectar
¾ cup nonfat Lactaid milk

Snack:
197
calories

4 graham crackers
1 cup nonfat Lactaid milk

Lunch:
417
calories

3 ounces tuna (packed in
    water)
3 cold asparagus tips
1 dill pickle
1 whole-wheat pita bread
    pocket
1 tablespoon mayonnaise
1 cup decaffeinated tea or
    spring water

Snack:
187
calories

1 slice Zucchini-Carrot Bread
    (Freeze remaining)
1 tablespoon jam
½ cup vegetable juice

Dinner:
589
calories

Lemon Herb Turkey with
    Brown Rice
1 cup herbed stewed
    tomatoes

1 whole-wheat roll
1 tablespoon jam
½ cup fruit nectar

Snack:
105
calories

1 serving Grandma's Rice
Pudding

Total Daily Calories: 1,803

MENU PLANS: DAY 14

Breakfast:
301
calories

1 soft-boiled egg
1 honey-oat muffin (freeze
remaining)
1 pat margarine
½ cup diluted orange juice
(50/50 with water)
1 cup decaffeinated tea or
spring water

Snack:
225
calories

1 cup fruit-flavored lowfat
yogurt

Lunch:
403
calories

Sonoma Chicken Salad with
Ginger Peach Dressing
1 whole-wheat roll
1 pat margarine
1 cup decaffeinated tea or
spring water

Snack:
200
calories

2 ounces skim mozzarella
cheese
4 Saltine crackers

Dinner:
619
calories

Shrimp-Rice Casserole
1 serving stuffed acorn
squash

1 pat margarine
1 plain honey-baked apple

Snack:
109
calories

2 canned peach halves (in fruit juice)

Total Daily Calories: 1,857

MENU PLANS: DAY 15

Breakfast:
295
calories

¾ cup ready-to-eat cereal
1 cup nonfat Lactaid milk
1 slice whole-wheat toast
1 pat margarine

Snack:
168
calories

½ cup fruit cocktail (packed in fruit juice)
4 graham crackers

Lunch:
379
calories

Herbed Oven-Fried Fish Fillets (freeze)
1 serving Oriental Oat Pilaf
1 cup French-cut green beans
1 cup decaffeinated tea or spring water

Snack:
277
calories

1/12 cake, angel food
1 cup nonfat Lactaid milk

Dinner:
610
calories

Turkey Pot Roast (freeze half for Day 18 dinner)
1 serving skillet corn bread
1 pat margarine
½ cup stewed tomatoes
½ cup pureed spinach
1 cup decaffeinated tea or spring water

Snack:
114
calories

½ cup fruit nectar
2 graham crackers

Total Daily Calories: 1,793

MENU PLANS: DAY 16

Breakfast:
308
calories

Mini Herbed Omelet (2
eggs)
½ toasted whole-wheat
English muffin
1 teaspoon jam
½ cup fruit nectar

Snack:
225
calories

1 cup fruited low-fat yogurt

Lunch:
403
calories

Sonoma Chicken Salad with
Ginger Peach Dressing
5 melba toast
1 pat margarine
1 cup decaffeinated tea or
spring water

Snack:
200
calories

½ cup vanilla pudding
2 graham crackers

Dinner:
592
calories

Tuna Soufflé
1 cup steamed sliced beets
1 whole-wheat roll
1 pat margarine
Maple Apple Crisp

Snack:
106
calories

Pumpkin-Apple Cream
Soup (freeze some for
later)

Total Daily Calories: 1,834

MENU PLANS: DAY 17

Breakfast:
277
calories

½ cup cooked cereal
4 canned apricots (packed in
    juice)
1 cup nonfat Lactaid milk
1 cup decaffeinated tea or
    spring water

Snack:
170
calories

½ bagel
1 tablespoon cream cheese
1 tablespoon jelly

Lunch:
406
calories

Tomato and cheese
    sandwich (2 ounces low-
    fat cheese; 2 slices whole-
    wheat bread; ½ tomato)
1 cup nonfat Lactaid milk
2 ginger snaps

Snack:
214
calories

1 serving Maple Apple Crisp
½ cup nonfat Lactaid milk

Dinner:
604
calories

Sonoma Chicken Salad with
    Ginger Peach Dressing
1 whole-wheat roll
1 pat margarine
½ cup sherbet
3 vanilla wafers

Snack:
100
calories

1 plain honey-baked apple

Total Daily Calories: 1,771

MENU PLANS: DAY 18

Breakfast:
286
calories

1 ready-to-eat whole-wheat
  waffle
½ cup applesauce
4 tablespoons ricotta cheese
  (part-skim)
1 cup decaffeinated tea

Snack:
200
calories

3 ounces salmon
4 wheat crackers
½ cup vegetable juice

Lunch:
411
calories

Pilgrim Pasta
1 whole-wheat roll
½ cup unsweetened
  applesauce
1 teaspoon jam
1 cup decaffeinated tea or
  spring water

Snack:
208
calories

2 ounces low-fat cheese or
  skim mozzarella
3 Ry-Krisp crackers

Dinner:
585
calories

Turkey Pot Roast
1 serving Skillet Corn Bread
½ cup stewed tomatoes
1 cup decaffeinated tea or
  spring water

Snack:
106
calories

1 serving Pumpkin-Apple
  Cream Soup

Total Daily Calories: 1,753

MENU PLANS: DAY 19

Breakfast:
319
calories

1 poached egg
½ cup tomato juice
½ whole-wheat English
    muffin
1 pat margarine
1 cup nonfat Lactaid milk

Snack:
168
calories

½ cup fruit cocktail (packed
    in fruit juice)
4 graham crackers

Lunch:
418
calories

1 turkey frankfurter
1 tablespoon ketchup
1 slice whole wheat bread
1 cup fruit-flavored low-fat
    yogurt

Snack:
200
calories

½ cup vanilla pudding
2 graham crackers

Dinner:
614
calories

Fish Florentine Wrap-Ups
1 cup brown rice
1 cup steamed yellow
    crookneck squash
¹⁄₁₂ cake, angel food

Snack:
87
calories

½ cup fruit nectar
1 graham cracker

Total Daily Calories: 1,806

MENU PLANS: DAY 20

Breakfast:
310
calories

½ cup cooked cereal
1 small peach, puréed
1 slice whole-wheat toast
½ cup nonfat Lactaid milk
1 pat margarine

Snack:
211
calories

1 plain baked apple
4 wheat crackers
2 teaspoons jelly

Lunch:
385
calories

1 cup low-fat cottage cheese
2 canned peach halves (in
    fruit juice)
5 melba toast
½ cup vegetable juice

Snack:
205
calories

1/12 cake, angel food
¾ cup nonfat Lactaid milk

Dinner:
609
calories

Pilgrim Pasta
1 whole-wheat roll
1 pat margarine
1 serving Indian Pudding
½ cup fruit nectar

Snack:
90 calories

½ cup vegetable juice
5 Saltine crackers

Total Daily Calories: 1,810

MENU PLANS: DAY 21

Breakfast:
290
calories

¾ cup ready-to-eat cereal
1 cup nonfat Lactaid milk
¾ cup blueberries
½ cup fruit nectar

Snack:
198
calories

1 serving Indian pudding
1 graham cracker

Lunch:
409
calories

Chicken Squash Rice Soup
1 whole-wheat roll
1 pat margarine
1 cup nonfat Lactaid milk

Snack:
201
calories

½ cup vanilla pudding
3 vanilla wafers

Dinner:
590
calories

Mediterranean Bouillabaise
1 serving Sweet Pilaf
½ cup French-cut green
   beans
¹⁄₁₂ cake, angel food
1 pat margarine

Snack:
106
calories

1 serving Pumpkin-Apple
   Cream Soup

Total Daily Calories: 1,794

MENU PLANS: DAY 22

Breakfast:
308
calories

2 Rice-and-Potato Pancakes
½ cup plain nonfat yogurt
½ cup applesauce
½ cup nonfat Lactaid milk

Snack:
192
calories

1 Honey-Oat Muffin
1 pat margarine

Lunch:
397
calories

1 serving Herbed Fish Fillets
¼ medium yam
1 Cornmeal Scone
1 pat margarine
1 cup decaffeinated tea or
  spring water

Snack:
216
calories

¹⁄₁₂ cake, angel food
1 cup nonfat Lactaid milk

Dinner:
598
calories

1 serving Chicken Dijon
  with Fettucine
1 serving Glazed Carrots
½ cup green peas
¾ cup canned fruit cocktail
  (packed in juice)
1 cup decaffeinated tea or
  spring water

Snack:
105
calories

1 serving Grandma's Rice
  Pudding

Total Daily Calories: 1,816

MENU PLANS: DAY 23

Breakfast:
301
calories

1 scrambled egg
1 Honey-Oat Muffin
1 pat margarine (unless
  some is used in making
  egg)
½ cup diluted orange juice
  (50/50 with water)

Snack:
197
calories

4 graham crackers
1 cup nonfat Lactaid milk

Lunch: 402 calories	2 Chicken Fajitas 4 stewed apricots ½ cup vegetable juice
Snack: 200 calories	2 ounces skim mozzarella 4 Saltine crackers

Dinner:
583
calories
	1 serving Turkey/Mushroom
	   Scallopini
	1 serving garden stuffing
	1 cup brown rice
	1 serving Meringued
	   Poached Pears

Snack: 106 calories	1 serving Pumpkin-Apple Cream Soup

Total Daily Calories: 1,789

MENU PLANS: DAY 24

Breakfast:
305
calories
	2-egg mini cheese omelet
	   made with 1 ounce skim
	   mozzarella
	1 slice whole-wheat toast
	1 cup decaffeinated tea

Snack: 288 calories	1 Cornmeal Scone 1 pat margarine 1 tablespoon jelly 1 cup fruit nectar

Lunch:
347
calories
	3 ounces ground turkey
	   patty (from skinless
	   breast)
	1 whole-wheat bun

1 teaspoon mustard
1 dill pickle
1 sliced tomato
1 fruit cup made with 2
   stewed plums and ½
   canned peach, sliced

Snack:
192
calories

1 Honey-Oat Muffin
1 pat margarine

Dinner:
476
calories

1 serving Halibut Chowder
3 steamed asparagus spears
1 cup stewed eggplant
1 pat margarine
1 serving Rice Spoon Bread
1 cup nonfat Lactaid milk

Snack:
109
calories

1 serving Meringued
   Poached Pears

Total Daily Calories: 1,717

MENU PLANS: DAY 25

Breakfast:
290
calories

¾ cup ready-to-eat cereal
1 cup nonfat Lactaid milk
¾ cup blueberries
½ cup fruit nectar

Snack:
192
calories

1 Honey-Oat Muffin
1 pat margarine

Lunch:
398
calories

1 serving Herbed Fish and
   Tomato Stew
1 Cornmeal Scone

1 pat margarine
¾ cup canned fruit cocktail
(packed in juice)
1 cup decaffeinated tea or
spring water

Snack:
200
calories

6 ginger snaps
1 cup nonfat Lactaid milk

Dinner:
585
calories

1 serving Roasted Game
Birds with Mushroom
Cream (includes ½ cup
rice)
½ cup French-cut green
beans
½ cup sherbet
1 vanilla wafer

Snack:
106
calories

1 serving Pumpkin-Apple
Cream Soup

Total Daily Calories: 1,771

MENU PLANS: DAY 26

Breakfast:
283
calories

½ cup cooked cereal
½ toasted bagel
1 tablespoon cream cheese
3 stewed plums
1 teaspoon jelly

Snack:
200
calories

2 ounces skim mozzarella
4 Saltine crackers

Lunch:
402
calories

2 Chicken Fajitas
4 stewed plums
½ cup vegetable juice

Snack:
216
calories

1/12 cake, angel food
1 cup nonfat Lactaid milk

Dinner:
590
calories

1 serving Flounder with
    Rosy Shrimp Sauce
1 cup stewed tomatoes and
    zucchini slices
1 Cornmeal Scone
1 pat margarine
¾ cup fruit nectar

Snack:
109
calories

1 serving Meringued
    Poached Pears

Total Daily Calories: 1,800

MENU PLANS: DAY 27

Breakfast:
305
calories

1 ready-to-eat whole-wheat
    waffle
2 canned peach halves
    (packed in juice)
1 tablespoon maple syrup
½ cup fruit nectar

Snack:
180
calories

1 cup fruit-flavored low-fat
    yogurt

Lunch:
391
calories

1 serving Lee Chou's Egg
    Drop Soup
4 Ry-Krisp crackers

¾ cup applesauce
1 cup decaffeinated tea or
   spring water

Snack:
192
calories

1 Honey-Oat Muffin
1 pat margarine

Dinner:
600
calories

1 serving Hunter's Style
   Chicken
1 whole-wheat dinner roll
1 pat margarine
1 cup nonfat Lactaid milk
1 serving Meringued
   Poached Pears

Snack:
105
calories

1 serving Grandma's Rice
   Pudding

Total Daily Calories: 1,773

MENU PLANS: DAY 28

Breakfast:
300
calories

1 Honey-Oat Muffin
1 pat margarine
1 teaspoon jelly
1 cup nonfat Lactaid milk
1 cup decaffeinated tea

Snack:
168
calories

1 Cornmeal Scone
1 pat margarine
1 tablespoon jelly

Lunch:
407
calories

1 serving Herbed Fish Fillets
1 Cornmeal Scone
1 pat margarine

2 canned pineapple rings
(packed in juice)
1 cup decaffeinated tea or
spring water

Snack:
187
calories

1 serving Pumpkin-Apple
Cream Soup
3 graham crackers

Dinner:
585
calories

1 serving Chicken
Ratatouille
½ cup brown rice
3 steamed asparagus spears
1 cup nonfat Lactaid milk
½ cup vanilla pudding

Snack:
109
calories

2 canned peach halves
(packed in juice)

Total Daily Calories: 1,756

MENU PLANS: DAY 29

Breakfast:
307
calories

1 scrambled egg (non-stick
pan, no butter)
¼ cup chopped spinach
1 slice whole-wheat toast
1 tablespoon jelly
1 cup nonfat Lactaid milk
1 cup decaffeinated tea

Snack:
187
calories

1 slice Zucchini-Carrot Bread
½ cup fruit nectar

Lunch:
417
calories

1 toasted tuna sandwich—2 slices whole-wheat toast; made with 3 ounces tuna (packed in water)
1 dill pickle
1 tablespoon mayonnaise
3 slices tomato
1 cup decaffeinated tea or spring water

Snack:
192
calories

1 Honey-Oat Muffin
1 tablespoon jelly

Dinner:
604
calories

1 serving Sonoma Chicken Salad with Ginger Peach Dressing
1 whole-wheat roll
1 tablespoon jelly
½ cup sherbet
3 vanilla wafers

Snack:
99
calories

2 graham crackers
½ cup nonfat Lactaid milk

Total Daily Calories: 1,806

MENU PLANS: DAY 30

Breakfast:
310
calories

½ cup cooked cereal
1 slice whole-wheat toast
1 pat margarine
3 stewed plums
½ cup nonfat Lactaid milk

163

Snack:
192
calories

1 Honey-Oat Muffin
1 pat margarine

Lunch:
385
calories

1 cup low-fat cottage cheese
2 canned peach halves
   (packed in juice)
5 melba toast
½ cup vegetable juice

Snack:
216
calories

1/12 cake, angel food
1 cup nonfat Lactaid milk

Dinner:
566
calories

1 serving Scallops à la
   Maison
1 Cornmeal Scone
1 pat margarine
1 cup steamed French-cut
   green beans
1 slice Zucchini-Carrot Bread
1 cup decaffeinated tea or
   spring water

Snack:
100
calories

1 honey-baked apple (plain
   baked)

Total Daily Calories: 1,769

CONCLUSION: NOW IT'S UP TO YOU

THE MIND IS A POWERFUL force. It works for you, but it can also work against you.

While the influence of one's mental state on a corresponding physical condition is becoming increasingly clear through medical research, it is already well established in the ailment we have come to know as irritable bowel syndrome. This book has presented several alternative ways in which to combine stress-reducing techniques with a nutritional program designed to ease the discomfort of I.B.S. symptoms and, to the extent possible, to minimize their recurrence.

But the real key to your success in enjoying a more relaxing and comfortable life lies in your ability to discipline yourself to take advantage of the help offered in these pages. The examples of other people who have learned to deal with this problem can serve as an incentive for you to take responsibility for your own well-being.

It will require important changes in your lifestyle and in your eating habits. Is it worth the effort? Ask yourself that question the next time you feel the approach of symptoms. The answer should come easily. Now set your mind to it.

REFERENCES

Almy, T.P., Abbot, F.K., Hinkle, L.E. 1950. Alterations in colonic function in man under stress. Hypomotility of the sigmoid colon and its relation to the mechanism of functional diarrhea. *Gastroenterology.*

American Digestive Disease Society. Spring/Summer 1986. Facing Facts: New Perspectives on IBS. *Living Healthy* 7:2–3.

American Digestive Disease Society. Winter 1986. Coping With Stress. *Living Healthy* 7:1.

Beech, Burns, and Sheffield. 1982. *A Behavioral Approach to the Management of Stress.* New York: John Wiley & Sons.

Bentley, S.J., Peason, D.J., Rix, K.J.B. August 1983. Food Hypersensitivity in Irritable Bowel Syndrome. *The Lancet.*

Bieliauskas, L. 1982. *Stress and its Relationship to Health and Illness.* Westview Press.

Brown, B. 1984. *Between Health and Illness.* Boston: Houghton Mifflin.

Burkitt, D.P., Walker, A.R.P., Painter, N.S. 1972. Effect of dietary fibre on stools and transit times and its role in the equation of disease. *The Lancet.*

Buttram, H.E. June 1986. Irritable Bowel Syndrome—Part I: Causes and Pathogenesis. *Clymer Health Clinic Health Report* 6:6.

Cann, P.A., Read, N.W., Holdsworth, C.D. 1984. What is the Benefit of Coarse Wheat Bran in Patients with Irritable Bowel Syndrome? *Gut.*

Charleston, E., Nathan, R. 1985. *Stress Management.* New York: Atheneum.

Chin, D., Milhorn, H.T., Robbins, J.G. 1985. Irritable Bowel Syndrome. *The Journal of Family Practice* 20:2.

Christensen, J. 1975. Myoelectrical control of the colon. *Gastroenterology.*

Cousins, Norman. 1979. *Anatomy of an Illness—as Perceived by the Patient: Reflections on Healing and Regeneration.* New York: W. W. Norton & Company.

Cress, G.A., Wilcott, R.C. 1982. Activity-Stress-Induced Pathology in the Colon and Rectum of the Rat. *Physiology and Behavior* 28.

Cummings, J.H. November 1984. Constipation, Dietary Fibre, and the Control of Large Bowel Function. *Postgraduate Medical Journal.*

Dinoso, V.P., Murthy, S.N.S., Goldstein, J., Rosner, B. 1983. Basal motility activity of the distal colon: A reappraisal. *Gastroenterology.*

Drossman, D.A., Sandler, R.S., McKee, D.C., Lovitz, A.J. 1982–83. Bowel Patterns Among Subjects Not Seeking Health Care. *Gastroenterology.*

Gindes, Bernard C. 1951. *New Concepts of Hypnosis: Theories, Techniques and Practical Applications.* Los Angeles: Melvin Powers Wilshire Book Company.

Jones, V.A., McLaughlin, P., Shorthouse, M., Workman, E., Hunter, J.O. November 1982. Food Intolerance: A Major Factor in the Pathogenesis of Irritable Bowel Syndrome. *The Lancet.*

Kruis, W., Thieme, C.H., Weinzierl, M., et al. 1984. A diagonistic score for the irritable bowel syndrome. *Gastroenterology* 87:1–7.

Levinson, S., Bhasker, M., Gibson, T.R., Morin, R., Snape, Jr., W.J. January 1985. Comparison of Intraluminal and Intravenous Mediators of Colonic Response to Eating. *Digestive Disease and Sciences* 30:1.

Manning, A.P., Thompson, W.G., Heaton, K.W., Morris,

A.F. 1978. Towards positive diagnosis of the irritable bowel. *British Medical Journal.*

Narducci, F., Snape, Jr., W.J., Battle, W.M., London, R.I., Cohen, S. January 1985. Increased Colonic Motility During Exposure to a Stressful Situation. *Digestive Diseases and Sciences* 30:1.

Neff, D.F., Blanchard, E.B. April 12–17, 1985. The Use of Relaxation and Biofeedback in the Treatment of Irritable Bowel Syndrome. *Proceedings of Biofeedback Society of America, Sixteenth Annual Meeting.*

Read, N.W., Krejs, G.J. Read, M.G., Santa Ana, C.A., Morawsky, G., Fortrand, J.S. 1980. Chronic diarrhea of unknown origin. *Gastroenterology.*

Richter, J.E. November/December 1985. Colonic Motility in IBS. *Practical Gastroenterology.*

Ritchie, J. 1966. Pain from distension of the pelvic colon by inflating a balloon in the irritable bowel syndrome. *Gut.*

Sandler, R.S., Drossman, D.A., Nathan, R.P., McKee, D.C. 1984. Symptom Complaints and Health Care Seeking Behavior in Subjects with Bowel Dysfunction. *Gastroenterology* 87.

Sarna, S.K., Bardakjian, B.L., Waterfall, W.E., Lind, J.F. 1980. Human colonic electrical control activity. *Gastroenterology*

Schuster, M.M. 1989. Irritable Bowel Syndrome. *Gastrointestinal Disease: Pathophysiology, Diagnosis, Management.*

Snape, Jr., W.J., Wright, S.H., Battle, W.M., Cohen, S. 1979. The gastrocolic response: evidence for a neural mechanism. *Gastroenterology.*

Snape, Jr., W.J., Carlson, G.M., Matarazzo, S.A., Cohen, S. 1977. Evidence that abnormal myoelectrical activity produces colonic motor dysfunction in the irritable bowel syndrome. *Gastroenterology.*

Taylor, I., Darby, C., Hammond, P., Basu, P. 1978. Is there a myoelectrical abnormality in the irritable bowel syndrome? *Gut.*

Thompson, W.G. September/October 1985. Clinical Features of the Irritable Bowel Syndrome. *Practical Gastronenterology.*

Thompson, W.G., Heaton, K.W. 1980. Functional bowel disorders in apparently healthy people. *Gastroenterology.*

Thompson, W.G. 1984. The irritable bowel. *Gut.*

Thompson, W.G. 1979. *The Irritable Gut.* Baltimore: University Park Press.

Van Vogt, A.E. 1965. *The Hypnotism Handbook.* Alhambra: Borden Publishing Company.

Whitehead, W.E., Winget, C., Fedaravicius, A.S., Wooley, S., Blackwell, B. 1982. Learned illness behaviour in patients with irritable bowel syndrome and peptic ulcer. *Digestive Diseases and Sciences.*

Whitehead, W.E., Engel, B.J., Schuster, M.M. 1980. Irritable bowel syndrome. Physiological and psychological differences between diarrhea-predominant and constipation-predominant patients. *Digestive Diseases and Sciences.*

Wise, T.N., Cooper, J.N., Ahmed, S. 1982. The efficacy of group therapy for patients with irritable bowel syndrome. *Psychosomatics.*

ORGANIZATIONS

National Foundation for Ileitis & Colitis
National Headquarters
444 Park Avenue South
New York, New York 10016
(212) 685-3440

The Biofeedback Society of America
10200 West 44th Avenue
Wheat Ridge, Colorado 80033
(303) 422-8436

National Digestive Disease Information Clearing House
Box NDDIC
Bethesda, Maryland 20892
(301) 468–6344

American Institute of Hypnotherapy
1805 East Garry Street
Santa Ana, California 92705
(714) 261–6400

Index

Index

Index

Index

Index